An Amazing Journey to Health

A Vegetarian Cookbook and Manual

Compiled by:
Juanita Prince
B.S., Family Science and Nutrition
M.A., Education

TEACH Services, Inc.
www.TEACHServices.com

**PRINTED IN
THE UNITED STATES OF AMERICA**

World rights reserved. This book or any portion thereof may not be copied
or reproduced in any form or manner whatever, except as provided by law,
without the written permission of the publisher, except by a reviewer
who may quote brief passages in a review.

The author assumes full responsibility for the accuracy
of all facts and quotations as cited in this book.

This book was written to provide accurate and authoritative information
in regard to the subject matter covered. It is sold with the understanding
that the publisher is not engaged in giving legal, accounting, medical
or other professional advice. If legal advice or other professional
expert assistance is required, the reader should seek
a competent professional person.

Copyright © 2010 TEACH Services, Inc.
ISBN-13: 978-1-57258-643-7
Library of Congress Control Number: 2010932555

Other books by Juanita Prince:
Ethnic Pride in Vegetarian Cooking - ISBN # 0-9663883-0-5

Published by
TEACH Services, Inc.
www.TEACHServices.com

An Amazing Journey to Health
Offers Healthy Earth-friendly Recipes

The Amazing Journey, and Informational recipe book, draws attention to the importance of positive thinking. The goal is to decide independently how to make a lifestyle change for better healt.

Other valuable information draws ones attention to our American food chain, and how rapidly it has changed since the last century. This is alarming. We must learn how to make positive choices for better health. If we have not learned yet how to make better choices for better health, the future may be bleak for us and we will have to face the consequences.

The book also provides wholesome healthy recipes that are earth balanced. Recipes that are low in cholesterol, fats, Tran's fatty acid, foods that are process free, does not contain dairy, and is GMO free. This book also transcends to a section of foods that helps to build the immune system. These healing foods provide a more natural therapeutic resistance to colds, flu like symptoms and other illnesses. Keeping the immune system in tact is what counts.

Dedication

This book is dedicated to my wonderful sister Eddie Mae Foster and my daughter Michelle Burrow. Eddie Mae's nursing career was rewarding. However, even more than the education she received, her desire was to work hard to serve others. Her work was her life, and she lived what she taught. She made a difference by encouraging her patients that they must be in control of their health. She taught that a healthy lifestyle is a choice, and not something you acquire by chance.

Michelle was a journalist when she married and had five children. By studying a wide variety of sources about proper nutrition, she educated herself completely about the details of good health. She dedicated herself to bring up her five children in a healthy environment. Her concern was that their meals were prepared carefully and with balanced nutrition.

Eddie Mae and Michelle are outstanding examples of active women in the community who live what they believe and help educate everyone they meet to live a better, longer, more stress-free, life through proper nutrition.

Foreword

Handicap and special needs children, always have been in my concerns. I have worked with them, and have counseled with their families a number of years, and one of the key components of services for these children is that good nutrition is essential, as should be true for all of us.

The message of health is, "unique", and not just unique for only one group of people. It has been scattered throughout the whole world, and there are people who are putting it into practice. In this regard, the mission statement and intent of this book, is to improve health through better nutrition, and to those interested in finding a better balanced relationship with their creator, combining the physical, mental and spiritual together.

Equally, the book serves as an informative handbook, or manual to bring about awareness of what has developed with our food chain in America today, and the directions that it is taking us. The book gives instructions on how to reverse these changes by making more selective and better food choices, for putting food into our mouths that will help us to maintain our health.

I have known Juanita seven years now, and whenever we talk, health and good nutrition is often brought up in our conversation. Juanita is very dedicated to health education.

In her "Amazing Journey to Health" there are patterns of ideas and suggestions that supports and helps to answer questions of inquiring minds about good health habits.

The book also helps to discriminate between foods that contribute to valuable health, and the foods that do not. I consider this book to be valuable and should be placed alongside your other health book.

Dr. Alfred Lewis, Ed.D

•••

Time brings about a change in our lives, and at such times, the health issue can begin to play a major role of interest in our lives. We hear a lot about health insurance, and what the baby Boomers of today are doing to survive the uncertain times that we live in.

Doctors play a major role in most of our lives and they can be helpful, but there is something that we can do for ourselves also by using prevention to lessen poor health habits, and learn how to support our immune system, by helping to build it up with powerful nutrition.

Today, because of the media and a wealth of information that is before us, we find a great source of information on diet and health. Therefore the doors are open to begin learning how to confront and prevent some of the health issues that may confront us.

Juanita Prince, a health educator for many years, has been very active and supportive of health programs. I got to know her through the CHIP program, where she acted as regional director for Spokane Washington for several years. CHIP is a Heart health program founded by Dr. Hans Diehl from Loma Linda, California.

With her back ground experience, teaching nutrition in schools and researching, she has now put together her second cookbook and manual. With a heartfelt desire, she wants others to be knowledgeable about the benefits and values of good nutrition.

I personally have had some association with Juanita, by participating in the programs that she took leadership in. She is dedicated to the health work. Her new book encourages and gives support to anyone that wants to make a life style change. Her book is also a guide that will teach and instruct how to select and put together healthy meals. I recommend her book for good nutrition.

Glenn H. Murphy, D.D.S.

Introduction

Such a time has come, to where individuals are asking health questions. Besides what their doctors are suggesting, they want to know more about themselves and what they can possibly do to feel better. It saddens me when I am approached by some individuals who say with sincerity, "I cannot go on like this, I need help! Can you help me? Visually, looking at their bodies tells the story. Both physically and mentally they are torn. They don't know what works, or where to begin.

Food scientists and nutritionists through the study of the plant kingdom, makes it very clear, that suffering everywhere prevails because it is largely due to popular errors in regard to diet. Diseases such as obesity, arteriosclerosis (hardening of the arteries), coronary heart disease, high blood pressure and cancer, are often reflected indicators of our life style and the foods we eat. I am truly convinced that a healthy life style makes a difference, with the experiences that I have had for myself. Simple prevention and God's protection has kept me from a lot of pain and suffering.

This book was written to help give back to society and anyone that has a will to learn, to know that the responsibility is theirs to live happy and peacefully in a well body. It takes only a few days journey, before one begins to feel the results of good nutrition. Reducing or eliminating processed and refined foods is important. Eating a whole food diet increased with fruits, vegetables, nuts/seeds and grains, becomes healing foods. The body needs healthy cells and enzymes to function properly.

Objectives

1. To boost the nutrient content of your diet by eating more grain rich foods.
2. To increase the intake of dark leafy greens, which is a plus to anyone who might have sugar diabetes.
3. To increase your intake of fruit: Blueberries for example, has been proven to have the highest level of antioxidants to protect cells from disease associated with aging, cancer and memory loss.
4. To stay away from genetically engineered foods.
5. To buy food from your local market. They support a clean environment.
6. To empower the diet daily to feed the cells with fresh green salads, live greens and fruit smoothies.
7. To use good nutrition to help heal whatever ails you.
8. To follow the natural laws of Health:
    Good Nutrition
    Exercise Daily
    Drink plenty of water
    Enough Sunshine within reason (advisable 15–20 minutes direct sunlight)
    Spend a few minutes each day breathing in fresh air
    Be temperate in all things
    Rest 7–8 hours a day
    Trust in God

Contents

Preparing the Body System for Cleansing 1

Exist to Live? Or Live to Exist? 13

Changes in Food Production 19

The Fundamentals of Building Good Health 23

The Benefits of Ingesting Raw Photochemicals 31

The Healthy Vegetarian Cuisine 41

    Scrumptious Salads 43

    Salad Dressings 53

    Tasty Soups and Stews 59

    Vegetables and Entrée Dishes 71

    Delightful Pasta Dishes 81

    Satisfying Rice Dishes 87

    Breads and Crackers 95

    Guiltless Desserts 103

Eating More Raw for a Healthier Life 115

Juicing for Life 125

Dairy Alternatives 131

Homeward Bound Dietary Plan 143

Herbal Seasonings 149

Terms, Definitions and Resources 155

Index 161

Preparing the Body System for Cleansing

Are We Thinking Clearly?

Often we have to accept the perplexities of life that comes our way, but it doesn't have to be that way. Today there is a lot of good healthy documented information that will help to support anyone who wants to have a healthy lifestyle

Staying healthy is a big issue, but one has to take the responsibility and do something about it. The degrading sick body will begin to send out messages when something is going wrong. Either you become serious about it and listen, or make excuses that everything is going to be fine.

Putting forth an effort to know and understand why our bodies are failing us seems to be too much to think about, so what can we do? We fall into a cycle that keeps repeating itself, with no success.

Having misconceived ideas causes misinterpretation of factual information that can be of some help to anyone who wants to rejuvenate their lives, and bring it back to a healthy balance.

A healthy life change requires planning. One has to make realistic goals, prioritizing in a clear step by step way.

Even though the goals are set, it still can be challenging, but they are possible to be conquered. Setting your rules and limitations that you are willing to abide by, with God's help, will help to keep you motivated with persistence and effort. It is exciting to know that within 2–3 weeks by staying on task with a healthy cuisine you will notice and feel the differences.

Motivation

The idea of doing something alone is often challenging and difficult to follow through with. The struggles are real, and are seen as big obstacles, that are almost impossible to surpass, but just think about it! Take yourself back to other goals you have accomplished in your life. It doesn't matter how small or big, or how long it took, you had the discipline to do it.

Support is very important. Seriously think of your needs for a support system. A social support can be your family, a friend or another outside group. Sharing your thoughts and feelings help to inspire to stay on task.

Once the most important decision of your life is made to take care of your health, the thought that you need to keep in mind, is how to continue to be motivated and let the life change become a natural part of you.

It is so easy to start a program and then after a few days become negligent, and fall away from your goal. It needs to be understood, that time is of value. Good things come to those that put the time in, and are determined to see the success. Therefore making that important choice to regain your health must be put into perspective.

Keep in mind that motivation is a natural aspect of human life. If we are to keep living, it becomes the key to productivity. It is innate from the beginning, proud parents watch their adorable babies struggle to pull themselves up from the floor to the table. There they stand with wobbly legs, as parents cheered them on with loving words. But the struggle did not end there. Other achievements had to be made in order to reach adulthood, and it continues.

This is why motivation is important. It helps to keep you on tract. Older people as well as young people can get back on their feet faster if they set goals. Motivation comes from within. There is an urge which moves us to action.

Maybe you are home most of the time, and do not have a five day job. Temptation still could be right there in your home, just a reach or more away from you.

Now is the time for you to clean house. Pull those addicting foods from your cupboards, refrigerator and pantry. Replace them with healing foods, designed to make you feel good, look good! And provide you with lots of energy.

Disease never comes without a cause. The way is prepared first, and then the disease is invited to come in, because the laws of health are disregarded.

When the abuse of health is carried so far, sickness is the result. The sufferer can often do for himself what no one else can do for him. The first thing to be done is to understand the character of the sickness and then go to work intelligently to move the cause.

Coping with Attitude

There is every reason to reform for the best in life, but God does not interfere. God has provided each of us with power to freely choose how we will live. God has given us tremendous power to shape our own future. Dr. Neil Nedley, M.D.

Every man has the opportunity to a great extent of making himself whatever he chooses to be. Our first destiny toward God and our fellow beings is of self-development. Every faculty with which the creator has endowed us with should be cultivated to the highest degree of perfection, that we may be able to do the greatest amount of good of which we are capable.

God can help us build up a character of solid worth to help us gain new strength, with every step we take can advance in more knowledge and wisdom. What a delightful difference, in the way we feel as we progress.

Facilities will improve by use; the more wisdom gained, the greater will be the capacity for acquiring. Ellen White.

Engaging in self management will require taking some steps. How you accomplish this is by checking out your attitude. Attitude makes all the difference in the way you act. Do you not recognize yourself as being the problem maker?

People, who will not make the effort to take step number one, will not take step number two. Turn eyes upon yourself, and discover that you are the only one that can change yourself. Talking to yourself is good, and listen, while you are talking. Change from fault, finding the changes that you can make.

Have faith. God is truly the author of our whole being. He will help to inspire us to true performance. It puts us in action and keeps us moving, to accomplish what we desire to do. Everyone has a different personality and our struggles are not the same, but there still is that desire that motivates each individual to do something.

Self interest always perks ones motivation, the desire comes from within. With that inner connection, can be a spiritual bond that connect us to our creator, which in addition can give us a deeper trust and faith to accomplish our goals. An additional bonus is that not only will we be contented with physical health, but we will also have created a new attitude with a peace of mind. Spirituality and Morality comes from within and are centered in the frontal lobe of the brain. The optimal choices for inspirational input seem to appeal to the spiritual and moral nature. Dr. Neal Nedley, M.D.

Food for the Mind

A healthy mind is a healthy body, bears a true statement. Testimony after testimony has been shared by many who have shared their experience of what a life change in eating healthy has done for them; they have more energy, and do not suffer from degenerative disease. They are off their medication with the approval from their doctor, after having a screening test done.

Food scientist and nutrition through research have proven that health foods not only benefit the body, but the mind too. The brain actually becomes healthier, when it is consistently provided with nutritional food.

Many neglect to think of how important it is to nourish their brain. Just like the heart, stomach and liver, the brain is an organ that is acutely sensitive to what we eat and drink to remain healthy. It needs different amounts of complex carbohydrates, essential fatty acids, amino acids, vitamins, minerals and water to help it function properly.

A sufficient balance of neurotransmitters are essential for good mental health, as they are influential in the feelings of contentment and anxiety, memory function and cognitive function.

Diseases never come without a cause. The way is prepared, and the disease is invited, because the laws of health are disregarded.

When the abuse of health is carried so far, sickness is the result. The sufferer can often do for himself, what no one else can do for him. The first thing to do is to analyze the cause of the sickness and then go to work intelligently to move the cause.

God has endowed us with a certain amount of vital force. He has also formed us with organs suited to maintain various functions of life, and he designed these organs to work together in harmony. If we carefully reserve the life forces, and keep the delicate mechanism of the body in order, the result is health, but if the vital force is to rapidly exhausted, the nervous system borrows powers to assist from its resources of strength, and when one organ is injured, others are affected. Nature bears much abuse without apparent resistance; she arouses and makes a determined effort to remove the effects of ill treatment she has suffered. Her effort to correct this condition is often manifested in fever and various other forms of sickness.

Foods that contain the following nutrients may help to improve the emotiona stability of the mind and body. Your diet may be deficient in the following foods.

Anxiety

Folic Acid
Green Leafy – spinach, lettuce, asparagus, beets, savory cabbage, bok choy, broccoli, green peas, fresh parsley, brussels sprouts, avocados and cauliflower.
Nuts and Seeds – peanuts, sesame seeds, hazel nuts, cashew nuts, walnuts.
Beans and Pulses – lentils, chick peas, black beans, kidney beans and pinto beans.
Fruit – oranges.

Magnesium

Vegetables – spinach, watercress, avocado, peppers, broccoli, brussels sprouts, green cabbage and watercress.
Nuts – almonds, brazil nuts, cashews, peanuts, macadamias, pistachios, walnuts and pecans.
Seeds – pumpkin, sunflower and poppy seeds.
Whole grains – oatmeal, wheat bran, long grain rice, buckwheat, barley and quinoa.
Fruit – bananas, kiwi, blackberries, strawberries, oranges and raisins.

Poor Concentration Attention

Vitamin B1

Whole grain – spelt bead oats, brown rice, barley and fresh pasta.
Pulses – lentils.
Vegetables – peppers, cabbage, broccoli, asparagus, romaine lettuce, mushrooms, spinach, watercress, green peas, aborigine and brussels sprouts.
Seeds – sunflower seeds and sesame seeds.
Nuts – brazil nuts, hazelnuts, pecans, pine nuts, pistachios and soya milk.

Depression

Vitamin B3

Whole grains – brown rice, rice bran and wheat germ.
Vegetables – broccoli mushrooms, cabbage, brussels sprouts, courgette and squash.
Nuts – peanuts and sunflower seeds.

Vitamin B6

Whole grains – brown rice, oats and bran barley.
Fruit – bananas and mango.
Vegetables – avocado, watercress, cauliflower, cabbage, peppers, squash, asparagus, bok choy and potato.
Beans – lima beans and soy beans.
Pulses – chick peas. Seeds-sunflower.

Vitamin C

Vegetables – red pepper, red cabbage, broccoli, brussels sprouts, cauliflower, kale, celery, squash, cabbage and watercress.
Fruit – strawberries, oranges, tangerines, kiwi, cantaloupe, papaya, cranberries and pineapple.

Folic Acid

Green Leafy Veggies – spinach, lettuce, asparagus, beets, savory cabbage, bok choy, broccoli, green peas, fresh parsley, brussels sprouts, avocados and cauliflower.
Nuts and Seeds – peanuts, sesame seeds, hazel nuts, cashew nuts and walnuts.

Beans and Pulses – lentils, chick peas, black beans, kidney beans and pinto beans.
Fruit – oranges.

Magnesium
Vegetables – spinach, watercress, avocado, peppers, broccoli, brussels sprouts, green cabbage, watercress.
Nuts – Almonds, brazil nuts, cashews, peanuts, macadamias, pistachios, walnuts, pecans. Seeds – pumpkin, sunflower seeds and poppy seeds.
Whole grains – oatmeal, wheat bran, long grain rice, buckwheat, barley and quinoa baked beans.
Fruit – bananas, kiwi, blackberries, strawberries, oranges and raisins.

Selenium
Whole grains – barley, rye, oats, long grain brown rice, wheat germ and brewer's yeast.
Vegetables – mushrooms, garlic, spinach.
Legumes – tofu.
Nuts – brazil nuts.
Seeds – mustard seed and sunflower seed.

Zinc
Nuts – cashews, walnuts and almonds.
Beans – chick peas, kidney beans, baked beans, lima beans.
Legumes – lentils.
Seeds – pumpkin seeds and sesame seeds.
Vegetables – spinach, mushrooms, squash, asparagus and broccoli.
Fruit – blackberries and kiwi.

Omega 3 Fatty Acid
Seeds – Flax seeds.
Nuts – walnuts.

Tryptophan
Nuts – almonds, pistachios, pecans, hazelnuts, peanuts and soy nuts.
Seeds – poppy, pumpkin, sesame.
Pulses and Beans – lentils, chick peas (hummus) kidney and lima beans.
Legumes – soya.
Vegetables – spinach, watercress and cabbage.
Whole grains – porridge oats, brown rice.
Fruits – bananas, pineapple, plums, dates, figs and prunes.

Tyrosine
Vegetables – avocados, green beans, tofu, miso soup, soy sauce, spinach and yeast extract.
Fruit – bananas, canned figs, plums, raisins, tomatoes and prunes.

GABA
Whole grains

Poor Memory

Vitamin B5
Whole grains – oatmeal, brown rice, wheat, bran and brown bread.
Fruits – watermelon, blackberries, lemons, raspberries and strawberries.
Vegetables – broccoli, watercress, cauliflower, alfalfa sprouts, peas, carrot, celery avocado, sweet potato and mushrooms.
Legumes – broad beans. Pulses – chick peas.

Vitamin B6
Whole grains – brown rice, oat, bran and barley.
Fruit – bananas and mango.
Vegetables – avocado, watercress, cauliflower, cabbage, peppers, squash, asparagus, bok choy and potato.
Beans – lima beans and soy beans.
Pulses – chick peas.
Seeds – sunflower seeds.

Vitamin B12
Nutritional yeast Flakes (Red Star®)

Omega 3 Fatty Acid
Seeds – flax.
Nuts – walnuts.

Irritability

Vitamin B6
Whole grains – brown rice, oats, bran and barley.
Fruit – bananas and mango.
Vegetables –avocado, watercress, cauliflower, cabbage, peppers, squash, asparagus, bok choy and potato.
Pulses and Beans – lima beans, soy beans and chick peas.
Seeds – sunflower seeds.

Magnesium
Vegetables – spinach, watercress, avocado, peppers, broccoli, brussels sprouts, green cabbage and watercress.
Nuts – almonds, brazil nuts, cashews, peanuts, macadamias, pistachios, walnuts and pecans.
Seeds – pumpkin, sunflower and poppy.
Whole Grains – oatmeal, wheat bran, long grain rice, buckwheat, barley, quinoa baked beans.
Fruit – bananas, kiwi, blackberries, strawberries, oranges and raisins.

Selenium
Whole grains – wheat germ and brewer's yeast.
Vegetables – mushrooms, garlic and spinach.
Legumes – tofu.
Nuts – brazil nuts.
Whole Grains – barley, rye, oats and long grain brown rice.
Seeds – mustard and sunflower.

Stress

Vitamin B6
Whole grains – brown rice, oats, bran and barley.
Fruit – bananas and mango.
Vegetables – avocado, watercress, bok choy and potato.
Beans – lima beans and soy beans.
Pulses – chick peas.
Seeds – sunflower seeds.

Vitamin B3
Whole Grains – brown rice, rice bran and wheat germ.
Vegetables – broccoli, mushrooms, cabbage, brussels sprouts, courgette and squash.
Nuts – peanuts.
Seeds – sunflower seeds.

Magnesium
Vegetables – spinach, watercress, avocado, peppers, broccoli, brussels sprouts and green cabbage.
Nuts – almonds, brazil nuts, cashews, peanuts, macadamias, pistachios, walnuts and pecans.
Seeds – pumpkin, sunflower and poppy.
Whole Grains – oatmeal, wheat bran, long grain rice, buckwheat, barley and quinoa baked beans.
Fruit – bananas, kiwi, blackberries, strawberries, oranges and raisins.

Confusion

Vitamin B12
The body carries a small lifetime source of B12. Red Star® nutritional yeast is high in B12. Sea vegetables are questionable.

Zinc
Nuts – cashews, walnuts and almonds.
Pulses – chick peas, kidney beans, baked beans and lima beans.
Legumes – lentils.
Seeds – pumpkin and sesame.
Vegetables – spinach, mushrooms, squash, asparagus and broccoli.
Fruit – blackberries and kiwi.

Insomnia

Magnesium
Vegetables – spinach, watercress, avocado, peppers, broccoli, brussels sprouts and green cabbage.
Nuts – Almonds, brazil nuts, cashews, peanuts, macadamias, pistachios, walnuts and pecans.
Seeds – pumpkin, sunflower and poppy.
Whole Grains – oatmeal, wheat bran, long grain rice, buckwheat, barley and quinoa.
Legumes – baked beans.
Fruit –bananas, kiwi, blackberries, strawberries, oranges and raisins.

Blank Mind

Zinc
Nuts – cashews, walnuts and almonds.
Pulses – baked beans, chick peas, lima beans and kidney beans.
Vegetables – spinach, mushrooms, squash, asparagus and broccoli.
Fruit – blackberries, kiwi.
Legumes – lentils.
Seeds – pumpkin and sesame.

Vitamin C
Fresh Fruit – cantaloupe, cranberries, kiwi, oranges, papaya, pineapple, strawberries and tangerines.
Green Leafy Veggies – broccoli, brussels sprouts, cabbage, cauliflower, celery, kale, red peppers, red cabbage, squash, watercress.

Folic Acid
Beans and Pulses – black beans, chick peas, kidney beans, lentils and pinto beans.

Fruit – oranges.
Green Leafy Veggies – asparagus, avocados, beets, bok choy, broccoli, brussels sprouts, cauliflower, fresh parsley, green peas, lettuce, savoy cabbage, spinach.
Nuts and Seeds – cashews, hazel nuts, peanuts, sesame seeds and walnuts.

Magnesium
Fruit – bananas, blackberries, kiwi, oranges, raisins.
Green Leafy Veggies – avocados, broccoli, brussels sprouts, green cabbage, peppers, spinach and watercress.
Legumes – baked beans.
Nuts – almonds, brazil nuts, cashews, macadamias, peanuts, pecans, pistachios and walnuts.
Seeds – poppy seeds, pumpkin and sunflower.
Whole Grains – barley, buckwheat, long grain rice, oatmeal, quinoa and wheat bran.

Selenium
Green Leafy Veggies – garlic and spinach.
Legumes – tofu.
Nuts – brazil nuts.
Whole Grains – barley, brewer's yeast, long grain brown rice, oats, rye and wheat germ.
Seeds – sunflower.

Zinc
Fruit – blackberries and kiwi.
Green Leafy Veggies – asparagus, broccoli, spinach, squash.
Nuts – cashews, walnuts and almonds.
Beans and Pulses – baked beans, chick peas, kidney beans and lima beans.
Legumes – lentils.
Seeds – pumpkin and sesame.

Omega 3 Fatty Acid
Seeds – flax.
Nuts – walnuts.

Tryptophan
Fruits – bananas, dates, figs, pineapple, plums, prunes.
Green Leafy Veggies – cabbage, spinach and watercress.
Pulses – lentils and chick peas (hummus).
Legumes – kidney and lima beans.
Nuts – soya nuts, almonds, hazelnuts, peanuts, pecans, pistachios.
Seeds – poppy seeds, pumpkin seeds and sesame seeds.
Whole Grains – brown rice and porridge oats.

Tyrosine
Fruit – bananas, figs, plums, prunes, raisins and tomatoes.
Green Leafy Veggies – avocados, green beans, spinach and yeast extract.

Loss of Appetite

Zinc
Fruit – blackberries and kiwi.
Green Leafy Veggies – asparagus, broccoli, spinach and squash.
Nuts – cashews, walnuts and almonds.
Pulses – baked beans, chick peas, kidney beans, lima beans.
Legumes – lentils.
Seeds – pumpkin and sesame.

Lack of Motivation

Zinc
Fruit – blackberries and kiwi.
Green Leafy Veggies – asparagus, broccoli, spinach and squash.
Nuts – cashews, walnuts and almonds.
Pulses – baked beans, chick peas, kidney beans and lima beans.
Legumes – lentils.
Seeds – pumpkin and sesame.

Tyrosine
Fruit – bananas, figs, plums, prunes, raisins and tomatoes.
Green Leafy Veggies – avocados, green beans, spinach and yeast extract.

Exist to Live?
Or Live to Exist?

Comfort Foods and Food Cravings

Regardless of whether you are, home, away from home or on the job, temptation can still be right there before you, just a reach or two away. If it is in your home, now is the time for you to clean house. Pull those addicting foods from you cupboards, refrigerator and pantry. Replace them with healing foods, designed to make you look good! Feel good! And provide you with lots energy. If you are away from home, it may be a good idea to think about preparing a lunch, or healthy snack while you are out, unless you can make good choices when eating out.

Disease never comes without a cause. The way is prepared first, and then the disease is invited to come in, because the laws of health are disregarded.

When the abuse of health is carried so far, sickness is the result. The sufferer can often do for himself what no one else can do for him. The first thing to be done is to understand the character of the sickness and then go to work intelligently to move the cause.

How to Break the Craving Habit

1. 'Self' talk. Ask yourself the question "Is eating this food an emotional clutch for me?"
2. What are my feelings before I started to indulge?
3. Am I suppressing lots of anger, sadness or frustration?
4. Am I edgy, irritable and restless?

True, comfort foods can sooth you and make you feel a little better, but it won't change your state of mind. It will just make you gain more weight, and could cause you to develop other serious problems.

Some rules for helping to break the habit are:

1. Keep a diary; note the feelings and emotion that prompt you to reach for the pastry.
2. Recognize and acknowledge what it is you're feeling. Work it out why you want to eat these kinds of foods, and then ask God to help you trace the roots and find out what you need to do.
3. Taking steps to resolve the problem may not be easy, but it is possible to do something. Even the smallest steps are in the right direction.
4. We all may have different reasons lying beneath the surface for being dependant on comfort foods. An example could be you are angry, and you may be producing a lot of excess adrenalin and stress hormones, go for a walk, a run, talk to someone in the family, or a friend.
5. Slowly try to wear yourself off your dependence on food, by making yourself wait 10 minutes before you eat. Each day add on another five minutes. Mean while implement your substitute activities. Go for a walk, ride a bike, listen to some inspirational music.
6. Once you recognize what changes you need to make, make new friends, get involved in community activities, go to the gym, enroll in school and take a favorite class, and go to church for spiritual support.

7. Remember it is about making small changes, step by step. Once this is accomplished, keep in mind that you will no longer have to turn to comfort foods. You have closed the door to old habits.

Foods such as white bread, ice cream, pastries, chocolates and drinks, such as tea and coffee induce an instant high because they make a rise in the blood sugar level. Quote Alex Kirchen, Nutritionist Laboratory Health Club London. This affects the nervous system and the brain, which rely on a continuous supply of blood sugar, or glucose for healthy function. The down side is that, because the blood sugar level shoots up so quickly, your body secretes too much insulin to compensate and so the effect is short-lived. Afterwards blood sugar levels drop even lower. This makes you crave even more for food."

To break out of this pattern, the solution is to keep the blood sugar steady throughout the day. Kirchen recommends, cutting down on foods that provoke this reaction that is any food that makes you crave even more food.

One in 10 people are addicted to food in the same way others are addicted to alcohol. The problem is the same with any addiction. An intense obsession with food leads to constant cravings. Most food addicts tend to be overweight. Which is bad for their long term health. So what triggers an addiction to food? Dr. Robert Lefever, an addiction expert, explains that in some people, craving originates from a defect in the mood center of the brain. Certain messages are transmitted from one cell to the next.

Some people are born like that, in the same way that some people are genetically predisposed to alcoholism. Eating the wrong foods make symptoms much worse, as it triggers more cravings. It is difficult for a person to deal with food addictions on their own. They should always seek professional help, to help them learn to substitute their addictive tendencies with other healthy behavior. An elimination diet is also important to reduce the intensity of cravings.

Healthy Foods that Promotes Comfort

Muscles weaken when in contact with certain types of food, because the energy field is disturbed, because of the communication between your brain and nervous system. The simple way to explain this is that muscles provide instant biofeedback when your brain is preoccupied with a food it doesn't like, then it momentarily forgets about the muscle.

It is wise not to eliminate any food, instead list foods that are suspects, and then get a professional diagnosis. Instead of reaching for foods that jeopardize us, we need to educate ourselves to find out what the healthy comfort foods are.

Cherries, rice and lentils, are some of the foods defined as wonderful foods that can have a positive effect on the body. Scientists at the Fuschr-Bosch institute of Clinical Pharmacology in Stutigart have found that these foods contain tiny amounts of valium-like chemicals, although the amounts are probably too minuscule to have a pharmaceutical effect. However, these foods are filling and nutritious and help keep cravings at bay.

Other calming foods are: celery, anise, cloves, cumin, fennel, ginger, sage, spearmint and parsley. These foods have a naturally calming effect, because they stimulate the production of serotonin.

The benefits of photochemical extend beyond the botanical world. These potent plant compounds appear to guard the human body from disease in a variety of ways. According to research, many photochemical help the body to dispose of potentially hazardous substances, including carcinogens, and may protect DNA in cells from damage that can trigger a disease process Hippocrates was purported as saying, "Let food be thy medicine and medicine be thou food. Scientists say that he may have been on to something. Since that time science has proven that the food we eat can prevent and in some cases fight diseases.

There are a wide variety of foods and components in foods that our bodies are programmed to use to keep us healthy, and if we are sick to make us well again, says Steven G. Pratt, M. D. of Supper Foods.

Another great writer and Health Consultant accredited as an early pioneer, says, "Physical habits have a great deal to do with the success of every individual". The more careful you are in your diet, the more simple and unstipulated the food that sustains the body in its harmonious action, the more clearly will be our conception of duty. There needs to be a careful review of every habit, every practice lest a morbid condition of the body shall cast a cloud upon us, E.G, White

Changes in Food Production

Genetic Engineered Foods

Companies that produce the genetically modified foods are saying that it is safe, but many question the idea. They say that not enough is known about the product. It seems as if the adulterated products were here on the market, before more information was given about it. Even the labels on the cans and packages did not reveal the information needed to describe the contents. Some of the excuses used for creating the GM products, were that high yield crops could be produced. It would eliminate starvation of the poor, and could produce bigger profits, depending upon the audience.

The problem with this new science is that experiments in the new laboratory are too limited to provide conclusive results, even though thousands of experiments may be conducted.

Consumers say no to genetically modified foods, because of some of the flaws and failures that have occurred. Some known cases of Animal genes that were crossed with plant genes, caused abnormal growth to the animal, and food that was not fit to eat.

An arising chorus of scientists, academics and ethics, have been voicing an alarm at this exploding and largely uncharted technology.

Consumers also feel that GM will remove consumer's choice. Organic farming could be ruined, because of contamination. GM genes are dominant. They are inherited at the expense of non-GM genes when cross pollination occurs between GM and conventional species. Consumers have been protesting against this new science. It was not until recently, that modified varieties were separated from the rest of the crops, and that a demand of labels be placed on the products.

Even though we are alarmed and threaten with what food Scientist are doing in this new millennia, we must remember were we came from. Our creator perfectly blue printed individually genes for human and animals. A few years ago, people did not dream of patenting plants and animals. It was fundamentally immoral, to patent plant and animal material, and to take the human DNA and patent its products violates the integrity of life itself.

The creator chose for our first parents the surroundings, best adapted for their health and happiness. He did not place them in a palace, or surround them with artificial adornments and luxuries, that so many today are struggling to obtain. He placed them in close touch with nature and in close communication with the holy one of heaven.

Avoiding genetically modified foods can be done by doing the following:

1. Buy more organic foods, they are not allowed to contain GM ingredients.
2. Read the labels.
3. Let your manufacturers know that you have stopped eating your favorite food from them, until they have confirmed they have removed the GM Ingredients.
4. For gardening, buy product labels that say, "No genetically engineered ingredients."
5. Don't be caught in a trap, learn what the major genetically engineered crops are, such as soy, cotton, canola and corn. Other modified crops include some U.S. Zucchini and yellow squash, Hawaiian and papaya.
6. For gardening, ask questions about the soil you are buying.
7. All plant seeds should be 100 % organic, they should be certified organically grown in accor-

dance with the National organic standards and meet or exceed Federal germination requirements.
8. Oregon State is the certifying agent who states that we have complied with the organic food production act of 1990.
9. Preserving Heirloom and traditional varieties have endured because their time-tested value to generations of gardeners and farmers. The Heirloom and traditional varieties are known for their great taste and high nutrition.

The seed of change certified organic research what they sell. Each year their researches cultivate hundreds of varieties of plants under organic conditions, to make sure that what you buy will thrive in your organic garden.

Why Buy From a Local Market

For consumer and vegetarians who wish to avoid GMO ingredient in their food, there are 10 valuable reasons that they should know why it is important to buy from the local market. The food and drug administration has been very slow about classifying the alien genes as food additives and therefore does not require that they be listed actually on food labels.

The 10 reasons to buy local:

1. Local grown foods taste better.
2. Local produce is better for you.
3. Local food is GMO free.
4. Local food preserves genetic diversity.
5. Local food supports local farm families.
6. Local food builds community.
7. Local food preserves open spaces.
8. Local foods, many times are less expensive.
9. Local foods travel less distances to be delivered.
10. Local foods were bred as nature intended.

The Fundamentals of Building Good Health

Food as a Medicine

Buying poor quality food and getting it as cheap as possible, does not necessarily mean that you got a bargain, and that you are saving. Harmful foods can cause disorders. Many are suffering with poor health today; because of their neglect too buy good quality food. Therefore, they are spending more money by paying for doctor bills.

Fast food diets have now become designer foods, and then of course the genetically engineering foods are added with some of the foods. The composition of these foods are mixed with:

Coloring
Hydrogenated
GMO
Fortified
High Sodium
High sugar
High Fat

The fundamentals of building good health, is first to educate the mind. Know what is good for the body, and what is vital for health.

Think of food as a pharmacy, with a variety of good choices to choose from, each foods are unique, together and separately, in powered too carry its nutrients to where ever it is needed.

Foods can prevent and cure disease, but they can also cause the disease. The best diet does not include a little of everything, but one that avoids the harmful. Fighting back with foods is using nutrition that aids you.

There are an increasing number of recent scientific studies related to foods, proving that plant foods have healing powers. By using a method of chemical analysis, they have become more precise. It has been proven that vegetables, fruit, grains and legumes have two compounds that are not found in animal's origins, which are antioxidants and photochemical curative properties.

Many scientists are inquisitive about the origin and significance of these beneficial substances found only in vegetables.

The question is why do we need them for health? The answer is that we have continued to need them from the beginning of time. In the book of Genesis it tells us that man's diet was fruit, vegetables, grains nuts/and seeds.

Later because of the discontent and murmuring, the flesh pots of Egypt was permitted, however the animal foods was advised to be used under careful restriction.

As blockages in God's timeline plan for a healthy diet continues to be interfered with. Men will have to become independent and find wholesome quality foods for him.

Reading through the book of Genesis and Exodus, we find that diets constantly changed. <u>Six diets</u> now exist since the beginning of time.

    1. First Diet: Fruit of the trees from the garden Gen. 3:2
    2. Second Diet: Plant Life and herbs of the field Gen: 3:17, 18
    3. Third Diet: Manna from heaven – Like coriander seed Ex. 16:24, Ex. 16:31

4. Fourth Diet: Flesh – animal food Ex. 16:8, 12
5. Fifth Diet: (1940–2000)
   Processed Foods
   Food Additions
   Coloring
   Flavoring
   Saturated Fats
   Hydrogenated
   High Sodium
6. Sixth Diet:
   Controlled Crops
   Food Alteration
   Genetic Engineered Foods

After viewing and studying these diets, ask yourself three questions:

1. Which was the best diet?
2. What two diets were the purest?
3. Where were the two major blockages?

It has been gratifying over the years to witness through scientific study, a full substantiation of great principles and instructions that was given to us since the beginning of time. Clearly pointed out to us was the connection between the food we eat and our physical and spiritual welfare. God intends to bring his people back to live upon simple fruits, vegetable, and grain. God provided fruit in its natural state for our first parents. He is bringing them back to the diet originally given to man.

Food can be a medicine when proper foods are eaten. There should be temperance in eating. Food place on the table should be of good quality, full of nutrition.

Some feel that plants and vegetable foods possessed healing powers by chance. These vegetables according to reasoning evolved the capacity to synthesize precisely, those nutritional and healing substances that would be needed by humans long before humans existed.

We may also consider with less validity a rational alternative; that a superior being created man and women and provided them an ideal "fuel" vegetable food.

No matter what one may believe about origins, numerous scientific studies demonstrate that vegetable foods prepared, provides the best fuel for our "engine". They supply the energy necessary to function and the substances to slow down the "wear and tear" over the years, and help to prevent break down.

The Importance of Having Good Nutrition

In our fast paste changing world today, we have seen a difference in our food chain. We have process, altered and GMO foods. These foods do offer the benefits for a healthy body.

The human body needs various nutrients and minerals to operate. The only way this can be accomplished is by maintain a healthy diet, by eating a variety of whole foods, fresh fruits and vegetables. From these foods you will get the vitamins and minerals needed. These foods are necessary to the body for many different reasons. They are crucial for obtaining energy, helping your body grow, and repairing worn out tissues.

When one does not have a proper diet, you can note the difference in their appearance. The body may be overweight or under weight, sickly, pale skin, and having little energy.

Healthy nutrients, points to a better way of life. Keeping fit by exercising while maintaining a healthy nutritional plan, can result in higher levels of energy, self esteem and a generally better feeling of well-being.

Healthy nutrition should begin at home. Parents modeling healthful food behavior have a powerful influence on food intake and preference in their children, especially when they are young. As a provider, parents should have influence over the types and amount of food made available to their children. Research shows that a child's reference for certain foods is dependent on the foods availability in the home. For example children raised in homes where fruit and vegetables are readily available often report greater preferences for these foods.

Solving High Sodium Intake

Breaking the salt habit is not an easy thing to do. It is almost as normal as eating an American apple pie. Ask an American chef who has taken his time to balance the seasoning in a well prepared meal. One of the things many customers will do is to reach across the table for a salt shaker.

We say that we eat salt for taste, but are there other reasons for not needing so much of it? Salt and sodium, is an electrolyte that your body needs. Electrolytes are minerals that dissolve in water and can carry electrical charges. Pure water does not conduct electricity, but water containing salt does.

The three major electrolytes are sodium, potassium and chloride. Other electrolytes are magnesium, calcium, zinc, and many others in very small amounts, (called minerals). They are electrically charged so they can carry nutrients into and out of your cells. They also send messages along your nerves and help control your heartbeat.

The body needs potassium and sodium together, to keep the body healthy. They are closely linked. The body needs a lot of potassium inside and a lot of sodium in the fluid outside, to keep the balance. Potassium and sodium constantly move back and forth through the cell membrane.

Cells need the correct balance of potassium and salt. The ratio should be three parts potassium and one part sodium. If the intake of the sodium is too great, the body will become oversupplied with sodium, and the body will excretes more sodium. If the kidney cannot secrete it, it causes the vascular system to constrict; the body dilutes the extra cellular sodium in the body by increasing the fluid volume in the body. This creates fluid retention.

To prevent high blood pressure, the silent disease, it is important to lower your blood pressure by increasing your potassium intake and decreasing the sodium. Since there are often no warnings when the blood pressure is high, it is a good idea to check your blood pressure often, and also to check in with your care provider.

Sodium is part of our food supply, and we get it naturally from grains, nuts, fruits and vegetables. If we want to add more salt, we must have some guide lines to follow, to keep from over indulging. FDA proposed that guide lines should be put on packages.

They suggest that sodium free would be less than 5 mg per serving. To be on the safe side, it is recommended that most people should eat no more than 1–3 grams of sodium per day. This would equal to one-half to two-thirds teaspoon of table salt.

Twenty five percent of salt we eat comes from the shaker, and the rest of it comes from hidden salt in the processed foods. This much salt makes it hard to control our sodium intake.

Sources of processed food with hidden salt are the following:

Macaroni and Cheese
Pringles
Soups
Celery salt
Mustard
Ketchup
Steak sauces
Baking Powder
Baking Soda
Potato chips
Corn chips
Saccharin-flavored soda
Ready to eat cereals
Corn Beef
American cheese
Can Chili and Beans
V-8 Juice
Cheetos
Kentucky Fried Chicken
Canned Tomato Bisque
Sauces
Salt

Now, more than ever, is the time to read the labels on cans and packages when shopping. Look for low salt, or alternatives like herbal seasonings that will season your food.

Focus on the product's serving size. Makers of salty foods often try to hide the fact by providing information based on small serving sizes. Be aware and focused. Take serving size into account when you buy.

Buying in bulk eliminates the problems of hidden sodium. The best alternative is to eat an abundance of unrefined foods, by eating freely of fresh fruit, vegetables, grains and other natural foods.

A few steps to lower the sodium problem, is to add wholesome bulk food to your shopping list. Many of these foods can be found at farmers market, or health food stores, and prepared at home. For snacks, there is no reason to pick up processed candies or cookies. The bulk sections carry a nice variety of dried fruits and nuts.

A few items to add to your alternative list:

- Fresh vegetables
- Homemade soup
- Shredded wheat
- Puffed rice or wheat
- Oatmeal
- Grain cereals (such as quinoa, millet, buckwheat and etc.)
- Legumes
- Brown Rice
- Low-sodium, ready-to-eat cereals
- Caraway seeds
- Fresh green or red peppers
- Garlic
- Fresh Parsley
- Sesame
- Fresh Thyme
- Lemon and other fresh herbal spices
- Multi grain crackers or home made
- Pasta (made from whole wheat or vegetables)
- Fresh fruit juices and smoothies or home made

The Benefits of Ingesting Raw Photochemicals

Restoring the Value of Eating Raw

Superior health, energy and strength to enjoy life fully, is a question of what percentage of raw food we are eating. Are we at all aware of how much our intake should be?

Research has revealed that the quality of nutrients we put into our bodies determine the quality of our lives. Many people do not seem to think that food is directly determining their physical and mental performance. Sports trainers and Nutritionist understand that for a body to be healthy there must be a change in lifestyle. Once a healthy diet is established and put into daily practice with three to four weeks, a difference in your health can be felt.

The advantage of eating raw is that it has major nutritional advantages. Raw foods are alive with antioxidants, vitamins, and minerals. The media today in this fast moving world, are our biggest competitors, its strong influence has taken away independent thinking from us. Seeing enticing comfort foods seems to follow us around. It is advertised everywhere.

We seem to be unconscious, as the food change continues to experiment with our foods, and in a short time, we begin to develop the degenerated disease.

America still is dumping garbage in their stomachs, and diseases are still on the increase. People don't want advice about what they should eat or not eat. They resist changing their diet, because there is something that they don't want to give up. Actually it is the other way around, God intended that man would gain something of great value.

Eating too much cooked foods has fewer advantages. When you set heat to food, enzymes are destroyed by temperatures over 118 degrees. Some food enzymes may be destroyed with temperatures as little as 105 degrees. They may not even survive light streaming.

Healthy food should be 80% alkaline and 20% acid. For good health and humor, eating raw is always essential. Quote: Dr. Baroody Food Theory.

Juicing Enhances Life

The rewards of juicing are absolutely great! The quality cannot be surpassed. The juice from the fruit and vegetable are not adulterated with, sugars, flavor, spices and added water.

The benefits of juicing are many. It is an easy effective way of doing something good for your body. Juicing bypasses the process of digesting whole foods.

Although juicing has major health benefits, it is also important to maintain a diet of healthy food. Both support the other. Juicing is a wonderful tool that we can use to stay healthy.

Why Juicing?

Juicing is a wonderful way to get beneficial enzymes. There are thousands of plant chemicals that researchers are trying to isolate and study. The plant chemicals, known as photochemical, are the cutting edge of nutritional research, because it holds the keys to prevent some of the disease we face. The advantage of juicing to the fullest is to use a wide range of fruits and vegetables to ensure nutritional balance.

Some vegetables are more difficult to tolerate or metabolize. Start slowly and find combinations that are beneficial

Another good reason for juicing is that we don't eat enough fruits and vegetable. Each day it has been recommended that we eat five servings of vegetables and fruit each day.

Few people realize that common foods used in their diets, contain as many of the same properties as laboratory produced pharmaceutical drugs, but natural foods possesses the power to combat illness and prolong life.

A mere generation ago, the study of the healing virtue of food was entwined with folklore, but it was unscientific.

Today because of studies done in human nutrition laboratories is changing the ways people think. Because of these studies more than 150, done in the last decade, really prove that it is diet that makes the health difference.

Benefits of Juicing for Life

1. Body absorbs larger amounts of nutrients.
2. Easy way to get beneficial enzymes.
3. Increases metabolic rate.
4. Ensures sufficient amount of photochemicals for the body.
5. Obtains a sufficient amount of powerful nutrients
6. Other immune enhancing properties are concentrated in juices
7. Juicing can help accelerate recovery from illness.
8. With specific combinations, fruit and vegetables target particular conditions and improve or alleviate symptoms has anti aging benefits.
9. Concentration of antioxidants in juice combats damaging effects of free radicals in the body.
10. Keep the skin free from wrinkles, and muscles will tone, and will also slow the onset of age-related to diseases.

Vitamins, minerals, amino acids (protein) enzymes, carbohydrate, fasts, water and fiber are all essential components of a healing diet. Every one of these essential components can be found in raw fruits and vegetables. This is a claim that can be made for no other type of food then raw fruits and vegetables.

Our first duty toward God and our fellow beings is that of self development. Every faculty with which the creator has endowed us should be cultivated to the highest degree of perfection.

There is only one lease on life that is granted to us; and the inquiry with everyone should be, "How can I invest my powers", so that they may yield the greatest benefits.

We cannot afford too dwarf or cripple any function of the body or mind. As surely as we do this, we must suffer the consequences.

Sprouting Providing Vitamins and Minerals

Raw vegetables not cooked, increases better opportunities of having good health, because it provides vitamins and minerals in its natural state. These vegetables are very important because of the folic acid and Biotin Foacin. Other vegetables just as valuable provide "good' sources of (B1), (B2), (B5) and (B6). Other special vegetables called the cruciferous plants are cabbage, broccoli, brussels sprouts, kale and cauliflower may also prevent other types of cancer from developing.

The leafy green vegetable carries a high concentration of folic acid. Many nutritionists believe that foliate deficiency occurs when vegetables are boiled and the water is thrown away. The reason is because the foliate is water soluble. It is believed that folic acid is damaged to some degree by heat.

Sprouting is easy, and is inexpensive to do. The grains and seeds do not cost that much and they are available at most health food bulk stores.

The time involved is very minimal and the harvest time comes quickly for most sprouts. The introduction of live foods in the body is essential to restore and maintain vibrant health. Eating sprouts are a perfect way to achieve this. Guy Lacroix / Sound Healing.

Value of Eating Sprouts:

1. Increases enzymes potential
2. Aids the digestive and assimilation of your food
3. More overall energy
4. Rejuvenate
5. Lentil and mung beans are high in protein (Sprouts ready in 2–3 days)

*Almost any seed, grain or legume can be sprouted.

How to sprout

1. Use a wide mouth mason jar.
2. Place a mesh cloth or stainless steel screen in place of the lid.
3. Fill the jar about ¼ full.
4. Rinse a couple of times.
5. Then let sit nearly full of water over night (8–12 hours).
6. In the morning, rinse a couple of times again, drain and place the jar upside down on a 45 degree angle to drain for the rest of the time.
7. Thereafter rinse the jars twice a day. Always keep the same angle, until you see white sprouts – about ¼ inch of growth, or about the size of the sprout itself.
8. Now things are ready to harvest. Rinse one last time and drain, transfer into a plastic bag or glass container with a lid and put in refrigerator for storing,
9. They will last for a week. Occasionally rinse every two days.

*Some nuts can be soaked overnight, such as almonds, without requiring a full sprouting cycle. Soaking nuts can increase the nutrient content, and make them more digestible for the body.

The Benefits of Healing Foods

Apples	Pectin, vitamins C and numerous photochemical that may prevent heart disease and certain cancers and also alleviate symptoms of allergies and asthma.
Apricots	Carotenoids, specifically beta carotene an important antioxidant, although fresh apricots are even better
Artichokes	Contains severally restorative nutrient, used since ancient times as a digestive aid and for poor liver function. Research reveals that artichokes may also confer cholesterol lowing benefits.
Asparagus	Low in fat, and low in sodium, a super vegetable for those who are watching their weight. A nutrient dense super food, asparagus may prevent heart, cancer and certain birth defects.
Avocados	Creamy, luscious avocados are such a rich source of vitamins, minerals, healthful fats and photochemicals that the U.S. government has revised its nutrition guide lines to urge Americans to eat more of them.
Bananas	B6, tryptophan, may promote a state of mind, may ward off heart disease, strokes and certain gastrointestinal woes.
Beans	A nourishing and hearty source of no animal protein, beans may help to reduce LDL ('bad') cholesterol levels, stabilize blood sugar, and help control weight. They may also prevent certain types of birth defects and cancer.
Beets	Rich, sweet and earthy in flavor, these ruby-red root vegetables are highly nutritious and provide fiber, foliate potassium, and such photochemicals as anthocyanins and saponins.
Berries	Tiny powerhouses of nutrition, berries are bursting with healthy compounds, including foliate, fiber and photochemical, which may improve memory and reduce the risk for developing heart disease and cancer.
Broccoli	Is a super food, has high levels of photochemicals and their potential to mobilize the body's natural disease-fighting resources.
Cabbage	Related to bok choy and brussels sprouts. A nutrient-rich family and loaded with protective compounds. This member of the family may cut off cancer and heart diseases.

The Benefits of Ingesting Raw Photochemicals

Carrots — Provides a good amount of beta-carotenes, as well as a good amount of fiber. Consuming carrots may help to protect against heart disease, certain types of cancer, skin disorders, eye conditions, constipation and high cholesterol.

Celery — Researchers have found comfort compounds in celery; including those that may help lower blood pressure or reduce the risk of certain types of cancer.

Citrus Fruits — Have an abundance of vitamin C, potassium, pectin, and photochemicals that may benefit numerous conditions, including allergies, asthma, cancer and the common cold.

Greens — Kale, swiss chard, collards, beat, turnips and mustard greens, are packed with vitamins, minerals, fiber and arrayed with phytochemicals that may reduce heart disease risk, eye disease and certain types of cancer.

Corn — A good source of complex carbohydrate, fiber, and thiamin and may help to fight heart disease, certain cancers, macular degeneration and obesity.

Figs — May help to prevent such ailments as cardio vascular disease, premenstrual syndrome and hemorrhoids. Especially rich in minerals, fiber and (polyphones,) compounds that neutralize free radicals.

Flax Seeds — Regulate blood pressure, is for cell membrane health, and may have the ability to prevent heart disease by reducing the production of hormone like substances that lead to blood clotting. The insoluble fiber keeps the digestive system running smoothly and helps to prevent constipation. Lignin in the fiber may play a protective role against autoimmune disorders, such as lupus erythematosus, rheumatoid arthritis, as well as fibrocystic breasts and some hormone related cancers.

Garlic — Back as far as 1500 bc, ancient Egyptians recommended garlic for a host of ailments, including heart disease, wounds, tumors, parasites and headaches.

Grapes — Contains photochemicals that may help to reduce risk for heart disease, cancer and strokes. Studies also indicate grape juice and raisins are also rich in disease fighting compounds.

Kiwi fruit — Provides large amounts of vitamin C, endowed with phytochemicals, that helps to boost your immune system and may stave off certain eye conditions, cancer and heart disease.

Lentils — These low fat, protein-rich legumes offer substantial phytochemical power, foliate and an impressive, amount of fibers more than a quarter of which is the heart-healthy soluble type. They have decent amounts.

Amazing Journey to Health

Melons	From cantaloupe to water melon-may help prevent acne cardiovascular disease, certain cancers, respiratory illness and vision loss.
Nuts	Are an excellent source of cardio-protective amino acid, arginne and also offers vitamin B.
Olive Oil	Is rich in unique disease-fighting photochemicals. Vitamin E and mono unsaturated fat, helps to clear cholesterol from arteries. Reach also suggest that olive oil may manage diabetes, rheumatoid arthritis, stroke and breast and colon cancer.
Onions	Chives, leeks and scallions are noted for their powerful photochemicals and the helpful fiber which may protect against cancer, cardiovascular disease and contstipation.
Peas	Fresh, sweet garden peas are a good source of plant-based protein (plant-derived) from making them an excellent food for vegetarians. Peas may help to reduce the risk for developing certain cancers, depression, help cholesterol and macular degeneration.
Peppers	Sweet peppers and spicy chili peppers add color and zest to your favorite dish, while protecting against heart disease, vision and nasal congestion.
Plums	Juicy vividly colored plums and prunes (dried plums) are packed with disease-fighting
Prunes	Antioxidants, and natural sugars. Prunes and prune juice are natural choices for relieving constipation and boasting heart health.
Pomegranate	Is an apple-sized fruit packed with jewel-like clusters of crimson seeds. The pomegranate is touted as an anti aging fruit that may prevent denying of the arteries.
Potatoes	Served in its high-fiber skin is nourishing, satisfying source of healing compounds.
Rice	Is a staple ingredient in cuisines worldwide, rice is an important source of complex fiber, and essential nutrients and free of gluten. Rice is a natural choice for people with celiac disease or wheat gluten allergies.
Salad Greens	Elevates the fiber intake and antioxidant levels. Arugula, Chicory, dandelion greens, escarole, radicchio, and water- cress offers myriad nutrients and health benefit.
Seeds	Rich in heart healthy fats, pumpkin, sesame and sunflower seeds, process an enormous amount of photo nutrients that may protect against cancers, cardiovascular disease cataracts, chronic fatigue syndrome and macular degeneration.

Soy foods	The richest dietary source of photo estrogen soy foods-tofu, edamame, dried soy beans, soy milk, miso, tempeh-posses high quality plant protein, lots of soluble fiber and a wealth of photo nutrients.
Spinach	Is a great source of iron. It has tremendous wealth of disease-fighting arytenoids and photochemicals that team up with vitamins to help produce against cancer, high cholesterol and vision loss.
Super grain	Is an ancient high-protein food with healing properties, so called super grain-amaranth, buckwheat, teff and quinoa are filling and rich in fiber, B vitamins and nutrients.
Sweet Potato	Vibrantly colored with arytenoids and filled with fiber, sweet potatoes are one of the most nutrient-dense vegetable. These roots may help to prevent cancer, degenerative disease, depression and heart disease.
Tomatoes	Heartily indulged in rich photochemicals. The nutrients in the vegetable seem to work in concert to protect against cancer, particularly prostate cancer, clogged arteries and skin ailments.
Turnips	Earthy roots, with a sweet, smoky flavor, turnips including the yellow rutabaga, are surprisingly full of vitamins and some essentials amino acids, complex carbohydrates and add to the healing power of the cabbage relative.
Whole grains	The nutritious grain and bran layer of whole grain are packed with photochemicals and insoluble fiber. Whole grains- barley, oat, rye and wheat-are linked to a lower risk for cancer, cardiovascular disease and diabetes.
Winter Squash	Are a relative to acorn and butter squash, colorful and delicious vegetables that may help to prevent acne, heart disease, macular degeneration and weight gain.

The Healthy Vegetarian Cuisine

Scrumptious Salads

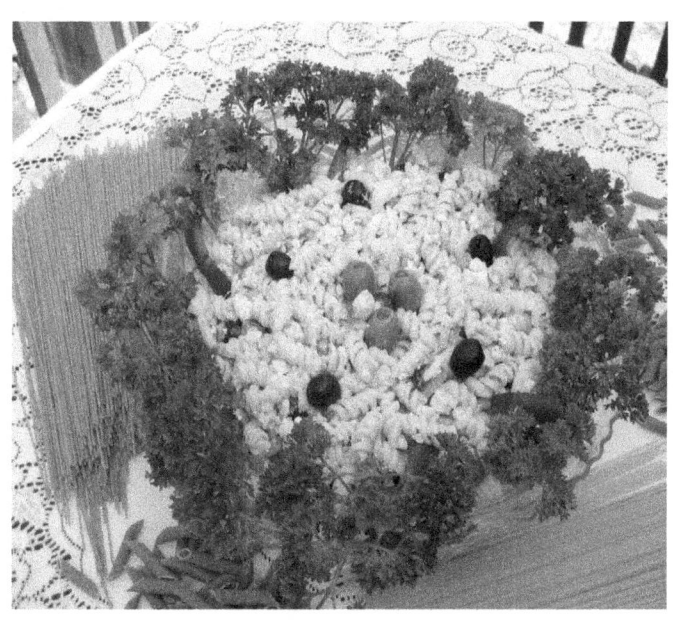

Black Bean Salad

2 cups fresh corn kernels from the cob
14 oz. black beans cooked, or canned (drain)
⅓ cup red pepper, diced
¾ cup cherry tomatoes, sliced
¼ cup green onions, chopped
2 tbsp olive oil
2 tsp fresh pressed garlic
2 tbsp lime juice
1 tbsp honey
¼ tsp sea salt
¼ cup fresh apple juice
1 jalapeno, seeded and finely minced
1 tsp ground cumin
1 head of romaine lettuce

Place black beans, red peppers, cherry tomatoes and green onions into a serving bowl.

Blend together lime juice, garlic juice, apple juice, honey, sea salt, minced jalapeno and cumin. Drizzle over salad, and toss to blend.

Break romaine off in bite size pieces. Serve the salad over a bed of lettuce.

Cabbage Salad

½ cup Chinese cabbage
¼ cup peanuts, chopped (can substitute with other nuts.)
1 tbsp sesame oil
1 tbsp honey
8 oz. firm tofu, cubed
1 tsp sea salt
1 tbsp Bragg Sprinkle Seasoning, (optional)
1 tbsp nutritional yeast, (optional)
2 cups carrots, shredded
2 cups cabbage, shredded
2 cups snow peas, slice in half length
½ cup green onions

Preheat oven to 350 degrees. Coat baking sheet with olive oil spray. Toss tofu with sesame seeds oil and honey in large bowl until well coated. Next sprinkle with Bragg Sprinkle Sseasoning or sea salt and nutritional yeast over the tofu. Spread cubes in single layers on prepared baking sheet for 30–35 minutes, or until brown. Turning over occasionally with spatula. Cool.

Combine Chinese cabbage, carrots, snow peas and onions in a bowl. Gently blend in tofu cubes.

Fruit Salad Mix

½ cup fresh peaches, sliced
½ cup fresh raspberries
1 cup cantaloupe, cubed
1 cup honeydew cubed
1 cup coconut cream or milk
⅛ tsp sea salt
1 ½ tbsp Eden® Agar flakes
1 tbsp maple syrup

In a sauce pan bring coconut milk, sea salt and Aga Aga flakes to a boil, stir occasionally. Reduce heat to low and simmer 2 minutes. Turn off heat.

Pour the liquid into a small square shallow dish. Set aside until jelled, then
Cut into ½ inch cubes.

Place the fruit into a serving bowl and mix in gently coconut cubes with the fruit in the bowl.

Garbanzo Bean Salad

2 ½ cups fresh small green beans, trimmed and cut in 1 inch pieces
1 15 oz. can of chick peas (or garbanzo), rinsed and drained
1 cup cherry tomatoes, cut in half
1 6 oz. can artichoke hearts, chopped
1 cup whole green olives
¼ cup red onions, slivered
¼ cup Italian parsley, finely chopped

Pour 1 inch of water into pot and boil. Reduce heat and add green beans. Let steam for 2–3 minutes until beans are crisp and fork tender. Cool, or dip into ice water to reserve color. Drain water off and set aside.

Place the green beans into a bowl with the other salad vegetables and toss together.

Tarragon Dressing

¼ cup fresh lemon juice
¼ cup fresh red apple
1 clove of garlic (or more if preferred)
¼ tsp sea salt
⅛ tsp cayenne pepper
¼ cup olive oil
2 tsp fresh tarragon, minced (or more if preferred)

Blend in electric mixer

Green Bean Salad

1 lb. small green beans, trimmed
4 cups fresh corn kernels, from the cob
1 medium red onion, chopped
¼ cup olive oil
1 tbsp honey
⅓ cup cilantro, chopped
2 tbsp lemon juice
½ jalapeno pepper, seeded and finely minced
1 tbsp lemon zest
1 tsp sea salt

Fill a medium pot half full of water, place over medium heat and let the water come to a boil. Place green beans in boiling water and let them cook for 5 minutes, or until tender, then remove beans from water.

Place beans ice cold water. When cool, drain off the cold water.

Place in a large serving bowl, green beans, corn, red onion, red peppers and cilantro. Add dressing and toss to blend.

Dressing

¼ cup olive oil
2 tbsp honey
2 tbsp lemon juice
1 tsp lemon zest

Green Vegetable Salad

2 medium size tomatoes, chopped
1 cucumber, diced
1 green onion, diced
⅓ cup olives, sliced
3 cups romaine lettuce, slivered
3 cups red leaf lettuce, slivered
2 large avocados, sliced

Place all prepared salad vegetables in a large serving bowl. Add all other vegetables. Toss and serve with ranch dressing.

Ranch dressing

1 cup silky tofu
2 tbsp water
¼ cup lemon juice
1 tbsp basil
1 ½ tsp onion power
1 tsp honey

Blend ingredients in a bowl, then pour into a dressing container.

Kidney Bean Avocado Salad

1 ½ cups kidney beans, cooked (drained) or organic canned kidney beans
⅓ cup red bell pepper, diced
⅓ cup celery, diced
¼ cup yellow onions, slivered
1 avocado, chopped
⅓ cup fresh corn
½ tsp sea salt or Bragg Sprinkle Seasoning

Over medium heat, add oil to skill. Add bell pepper, celery, onion and corn. Sauté for 2 minutes. Add sea salt or Bragg Sprinkle Seasoning, to taste.

Place vegetables from skillet into bowl. Add kidney beans and avocado to dish. Toss gently together. Add Dressing.

Dressing

¾ cup cilantro
½ cup fresh dill
½ cup fresh basil
2 tbsp fresh lemon juice
2 tbsp olive oil
2 tbsp honey or (another healthy sweetener if preferred)

Blend together well, then place in refrigerator to chill until read for use.

Potato Cucumber Salad

1 lb. Yukon Gold potatoes (or red potatoes), boiled and diced
⅓ cup tofu sour cream
⅜ oz. firm tofu, crumbled
2 tbsp fresh dill, chopped
1 cucumber, chopped
1 kosher pickle, minced (no vinegar)
2 tbsp kosher pickle juice (no vinegar)
¼ cup onions, chopped
¼ cup green olives
2–3 tsp veggie chik seasoning
¼ tsp Celtic Sea Salt®

Place chopped potatoes in large bowl. Add crumbled tofu, tofu sour cream and then blend together. Add all the remaining ingredients and mix. Cover bowl and then set in the refrigerator to chill until ready to serve.

Note. Bubbies® pickles are a kosher pickle without the vinegar

Tabbouleh

1 ¼ cup fine bulgur
¼ cup wild rice, cooked
3 tbsp lemon juice
2 tsp honey
1 tsp sea salt
1 ⅓ cup pistachios nuts, finely chopped
1 cup parsley, chopped
1 medium tomato, chopped
4 green onions, finely chopped
⅓ cup fresh mint, finely chopped
3 tbsp olive oil

Place bulgur in large bowl and add ⅓ cup boiling water. Let stand 5 minutes more until all liquid is absorbed.

Add rice and fluff mixture together. Stir in remaining ingredient and season with salt or natural herb spices.

Salad Dressings

Creamy Garlic and Onion Salad Dressing

1 cup silky tofu
2 tbsp parsley, minced
1 tbsp fresh lemon juice
2 cloves garlic, minced
1 tbsp honey
¼ tsp sea salt
¼ cup soy sour cream
1 tbsp onion, grated

Combine all ingredients into a blender. Blend until smooth. Cover and chill.

Italian Dressing

1 cup silky tofu
1 tbsp fresh lemon juice
2 cloves garlic, minced
3 dates
¼ tsp sea salt
⅛ tsp cayenne pepper
1 tbsp fresh basil leaves, minced

Blend in food blender for 2 minutes

Pimento Relish Dressing

½ cup silky tofu
2–3 tsp fresh lemon juice
1 small jar pimentos
2 tbsp healthy pickles, diced

Place tofu, lemon juice and pimentos in blender. Blend well. Put in bowl and add diced pickles.

Sesame Seed Dressing

1 small green onion, chopped
1 cup cucumbers, chopped
1 tbsp lemon juice
3 tbsp sesame seeds
¼ cup olives
½ tsp salt
1 tsp paprika
2 tsp honey

Whiz ingredients together. May be served with a cabbage salad.

Sour Cream Dressing

1 cup soy sour cream
3 tbsp fresh tarragon
2 tbsp fresh chives
1 tbsp lime juice
1 clove garlic
2 tsp honey
⅛ tsp sea salt

Combine all ingredients together in a blender, mix until smooth.

Thousand Island dressing

1 cup silk tofu
1 Serrano chili, seed and veined
1 roma tomato, chopped
2 tbsp green onions, chopped
2 tbsp celery
1 clove garlic
1 tsp honey
1 tsp paprika
¼ tsp sea salt

Place all ingredients into a blender and mix well.

Tomato Almond Dressing

¼ cup almond butter
⅓ cup tomato juice
2 tsp nutritional yeast (optional)
¼ cup sesame oil
salt to taste

Liquify tomato juice with almond butter. Slowly add the oil, beating till smooth.

Tasty Soups and Stews

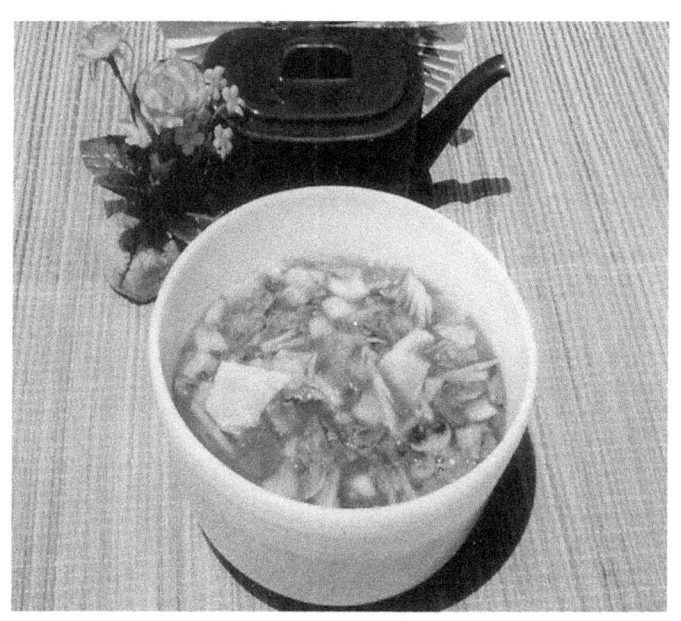

Black Bean Chili

1 lb. dried black beans
2 tbsp olive oil
1 cup soy baco bits
⅓ cup celery, chopped
1 large onion, chopped
2 carrots, finely chopped
1 Serrano chili, seeded and minced
1 tbsp veggie beef seasoning
2 tbsp chili powder
1 tbsp Spike® Seasoning
1 tsp salt
1 tsp cayenne pepper
8 Italian plum tomatoes, chopped
½ cup cilantro, chopped
2 cloves garlic, minced
1 tsp ground coriander
1 tbsp fresh lime juice
1 cup soy sour cream
Additional cilantro, minced for garnish
Additional tomato, chopped for garnish

Place beans in pot and cover with water to cover 3 inches over top. Let water come to a hard boil and then turn off. Cover beans and let set over night. Drain off water and rinse beans well. Cover beans and cook on medium for 1 hour, or until done.

Add olive oil and all other ingredients, except lime juice and sour cream. Mix sour cream and lime juice together and blend. In another bowl, combine tomatoes and cilantro. Ladle into bowls then add toppings.

Black French Lentil Soup

1 lb. French black lentils
5 cloves garlic, crushed
½ cup onions, chopped
1 red pepper, chopped
½ cup cabbage, chopped
1 cup fresh corn
1 tbsp fresh parsley, minced
⅓ cup celery, chopped
8 roma tomatoes, crushed
½ cup carrots, chopped
2 tbsp veggie chik seasoning, or more for taste
1 tsp sea salt

Place lentils in pot and cover with about 2 inches over the top of lentils. Cover pot, simmer and cook until desired tenderness.

Cabbage Corn Chowder

¼ cup TVP (soy textured protein)
1 onion, chopped
14 oz. fresh corn, or frozen
1 ½ cups yellow potatoes, cooked
½ red bell pepper, chopped
2 cups fresh cabbage, chopped
1 tbsp olive oil
3 cups soy milk
8 oz. coconut milk
1 tsp sea salt
1 tsp cayenne pepper
1 tbsp veggie chik seasoning

Cut corn off the cob, or use frozen corn. Place in a blender and process until smooth. Pour into a sauce pot. Place potatoes in a blender, add potatoes, soy milk and salt. Blend well. Add to sauce in pot.

Pour olive oil into a sauce pan and add green peppers, cabbage and sauté for three minutes. Blend with cayenne pepper and veggie chik seasoning. When tender, blend with sauce and add coconut milk. Cover pan and place on low heat. Let simmer for ten minutes, stirring at least 2–3 times.

Chili Pinto Beans

5 cups pinto beans, cooked and drain (save liquid, for if needed)
2 tbsp olive oil
2 large onions, chopped
4 oz. garlic, chopped
1 cup TVP (soy textured protein), soaked in 1 cup water
¼ cup masa harina, finely milled corn flour
10 large Italian plum tomatoes, chopped
¼ cup celery, chopped
4 tbsp chili powder
2 tbsp ground cumin
1 tsp oregano
1 tsp cayenne pepper
1 jalapeno pepper, seeded, deveined and chopped (optional)
1 fresh Serrano pepper, seeded, deveined and chopped (optional)
1 chipotle pepper, chopped (optional)

To remove the skin from the pepper, hold pepper over open flame and char on both sides. Place the pepper in a brown paper bag and close. Let sweat about 10 minutes. Skin should remove easily.

Put olive oil in a large pot over medium heat, add onions, garlic and celery. Drain water from TVP and add TVP to vegetables in pot and stir for one minute to blend. Add masa harina and blend in. Add remaining ingredients. Cover pot and simmer on low for 20 minutes.

Note: If chili needs more liquid, use liquid from beans that were drained.

Cream of Asparagus Soup

1 lb. fresh asparagus, trimmed and cut into 1 inch pieces
½ cup onions, chopped
1 tbsp olive oil
1 tbsp veggie chik seasoning
1 ½ cups soy milk
⅓ cup cashew nuts
2 tbsp pastry wheat flour
1 tsp sea salt
1 tsp herbal seasoning salt
½ tsp cayenne pepper
½ cup soy sour cream
1 tsp fresh lemon juice

Combine in blender soy milk and cashew nuts. Blend until smooth, add pastry wheat flour and blend again. Add soy sour cream and lemon juice. Pour mixture into a sauce pan over low heat and stir until it thickens.

Combine in a sauce pan, olive oil, asparagus, chopped onions, sea salt and herbal seasoning. Cover top. Simmer until vegetables are tender.

Combine cream sauce and vegetables together and blend.

Creamy Broccoli Chowder

10 oz. fresh broccoli, steamed and chopped
2 cups soy milk
16 oz. coconut milk
8 oz. tofu sour cream
1 medium onion, chopped
⅓ cup water
3 cups Yukon Gold potatoes, chopped
2 cups water
1 tbsp veggie chik seasoning
1 tsp sea salt

Place potatoes in sauce pan, cover with 2 cups water and cook until tender.

Place in sauce pot ⅓ cup water and onions. Sauté onions until tender. Then add broccoli, cook for 2 minutes while stirring. Add to pot soy milk, coconut milk, sour cream, potatoes, veggie chik seasoning and sea salt. Blend.

Cover pot and simmer chowder over low heat for 15 minutes.

Greek White Bean Soup

1 lb. large lima beans
1 large red onion, chopped
1 cup leeks, chopped white part only
2 tbsp veggie chik seasoning
1 tsp sea salt
1 tbsp nutritional yeast (optional)
½ tsp cayenne pepper
2 cups baby spinach
⅓ cup rice cheese or vegan cheddar cheese for garnish

Soak the lima beans in cold water for 2–4 hours. When they are wrinkled and splitting open, drain the water off the beans.

Place the beans in a deep heavy sauce pot. Add two cups of cold water. Cover and simmer the beans until they are soft, for 1 hour or until tender. Add salt and cayenne pepper. Pour olive oil in sauce pan, and add onions and leeks. Sauté 3 minutes. Add baby spinach. Take half the beans and puree in a blender, then add back to the pot. Add the sautéed vegetables and blend. Garnish with rice cheese.

Lentil Combo

3 cups French lentils, cooked
1 cup barley, cooked
¼ cup water
¼ cup olive oil
1 carrot, chopped
¼ cup celery, chopped
¼ cup onion, chopped
6 roma tomatoes, chopped
3 cloves garlic, minced
¼ cup tomato paste
1 Serrano chili, seeded, veined and minced
1 tsp sea salt
1 tbsp veggie chik seasoning
1 tbsp nutritional yeast (optional)

Place in sauce pan with olive oil over medium heat, add celery, onion and carrots. Sauté for two minutes or until vegetables are tender.

Add tomatoes, chili pepper, cilantro, garlic tomato paste, sea salt, nutritional yeast, cumin and veggie chik seasoning to vegetables in pan. Cover pan and simmer for 3 minutes.

Place lentils and barley together in a large pot, then add all the cooked vegetables. Cover pot and simmer on low, 10–15 minutes.

Northern Bean Soup

2 cups great northern beans
8 oz. tomato sauce
¼ cup nutritional yeast (optional)
1 large onion, chopped
1 tbsp vegetarian beef seasoning
1 tsp Celtic Sea Salt®
½ tsp cayenne pepper
3 cloves garlic, minced
2 cups Yukon gold or yellow potatoes, chopped
2 cups carrots, chopped
⅓ cup celery, chopped

Place beans in a medium size sauce pot and cover with water, about 2 inches over beans. Bring beans to a rapid boil for 2 minutes. Remove beans from heat. Cover and let stand for 1 hour.

Add tomato sauce, soy baco chips, onion and garlic to beans. Heat to boiling and then reduce heat. Cover and simmer for about 1 hour. Add potatoes, carrots, celery, vegetarian beef seasoning and sea salt, cover pot and continue to cook on low heat of 1 hour, or until vegetables are tender in soup.

Potato Vegetable Soup

3 cups water
2 Yukon gold potatoes, peeled and cubed (any potatoes could be used.)
3 stalk celery, chopped
2 large carrots, chopped
1 cup tiny green peas
½ cup onions, chopped
1 tbsp olive oil
8 oz. coconut milk
1 tsp salt
1 tbsp veggie chik seasoning
1 tbsp nutritional yeast (optional)

Pour water into a deep sauce pot, add potatoes, celery, onions and olive oil. Cover pot and Simmer on low heat for five minutes, or until vegetables are tender. Add green peas, coconut milk and seasonings. Stir vegetables. Place on low heat and let simmer for 15 minutes while stirring occasionally

Savory Chickpea Stew

2 tbsp olive oil
1 small onion, thinly sliced
3 cloves garlic, minced
14 oz. chick peas, cooked (or use canned chickpeas)
3 medium carrots, chopped
2 tsp ground cumin
1 tsp turmeric ground (optional)
1 tsp cayenne pepper
¼ cup cilantro leaves, minced
2 tsp honey
2 tbsp veggie chik seasoning
¼ tsp Celtic Sea Salt®
2 cups water

Heat oil in large skillet over medium heat. Add onions, garlic and chopped carrots. Sauté for 3 minutes. Stir in chickpeas, cumin, turmeric, cayenne pepper, cilantro and veggie chik seasoning. Add water and blend with mixture. Turn heat down to low, cover skillet with top and let stew simmer for 10–15 minutes more. Remove the top, and crush some of the chickpeas to create more sauce in the mixture. Cover skillet again and cook for five more minutes.

To top this dish off, serve with tofu sour cream.

Tomato Tofu Soup

2 tbsp olive oil
6 oz. firm tofu, drained and crumbled
1 tbsp veggie chik seasoning
1 tsp salt
1 cup red onions, chopped
1 tsp ginger, grated
1 tsp curry powder
1 tbsp fresh basil, minced
¼ tsp thyme
⅓ cup water
10 roma tomatoes, chopped and crushed
8 oz. tomato paste
1 tbsp honey
14 oz. coconut milk
2 tbsp nutritional yeast (optional)

Pour in sauce pot, olive oil and water. Place over heat and add ginger, curry powder, basil, thyme and onions. Cover pan and simmer for 3 minutes. Add crumbled tofu and blend in with seasoning. Simmer for 3 more minutes.

Add to sauce pot crushed tomatoes, tomato paste, honey, coconut milk and salt. Stir to blend all ingredients.

Divide the soup in two portions, blend each portion in a vita mix or food processor until smooth. Add both portions back into sauce pot, and serve.

Vegetables and Entrée Dishes

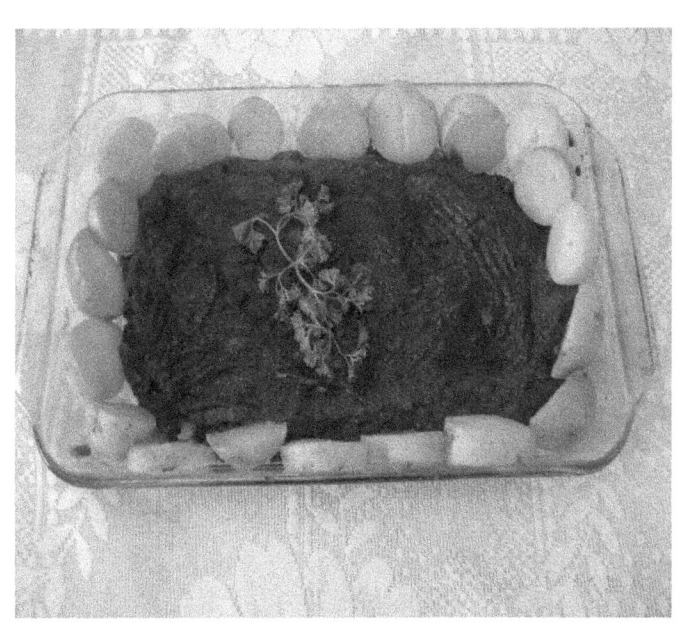

Asparagus with Cream Sauce

2 lbs. asparagus, (trim off rough edges on the bottom) wash
8 oz. block rice cheese, or vegan soy cheese
1 tbsp lemon juice, fresh
1 tsp sea salt
1–2 tbsp olive oil
⅓ cup onions, slivered
6 mushrooms, sliced
12 red bell peppers, cut in slices
2 tsp veggie chik Seasoning

Cut asparagus in thirds. Steam until fork tender. Do not overcook.
Place in blender coconut cream, rice cheese, lemon juice and sea salt.
Pour mixture from blender into sauce pan, stir until it begins to thicken.
Pour oil in sauce pan over medium heat, add onions, mushrooms and red
bell peppers. Sauté 2 minutes.

Place asparagus in casserole dish, top with sauce, cover the top with the onions, mushrooms, and bell peppers.

Broccoli Tofu Scramble

8 oz. tofu, crumbled
1 ½ cup fresh broccoli
2 cups water
⅓ cup onions, chopped
¼ cup red bell peppers, diced
3 cloves garlic, minced
⅓ cup block rice cheese, shredded
¼ tsp sea salt
2 tsp Bragg Liquid Aminos (optional)
1 tbsp veggie chik seasoning
dash cayenne pepper (optional)
2–3 tsp olive oil
¼ cup coconut milk

Add three cups of water to a pot. Let it heat to boiling, and then add broccoli. Sit in the hot water 3 minutes, then remove broccoli. When cooled, chop in small pieces

Put olive oil into a skillet over low heat, when warm add the onions, red bell pepper and garlic. Stir for two minutes, then add crumbled tofu, stir 2–3 minutes, then add broccoli. Add sea salt and amino, stir to blend, and then add coconut milk and shredded rice cheese. Cover skillet to let the cheese melt 1–2 minutes.

*Served with fresh sliced apples and toast.

Tip: Broccoli may be steamed or stir fried lightly.

Cheesy Broccoli

1 lb. fresh broccoli, steamed
½ cup coconut cream
4 oz. block or slice rice cheese, shredded
½ red bell pepper, chopped
¼ cup onions, chopped
2 tsp. soy baco bits

Place in blender coconut cream and rice cheese. Blend until smooth. Add red pepper, onion and salt.

Pour liquid ingredient from blender into a sauce pan, and place over low heat. Stir until it began to thicken.

Drain liquid from fresh broccoli, place in a casserole dish and cover with sauce.

Fancy Brussels Sprouts

1 ½ lbs. brussels sprouts
2 tsp veggie chik seasoning
1 tsp salt
1 tbsp olive oil
1 onion, chopped
1 green pepper, seeded and chopped
1 lb. tomatoes, chopped
2–3 cloves garlic, chopped
½ tsp fresh basil
1 tbsp honey (optional)
1 tbsp unbleached flour

Trim Brussels sprouts. Cut the bulbs in half. Wash them thoroughly.

Cook the sprouts in boiling hot water, until about tender. (10–12 minutes.)

Place the oil into a pan over moderate heat. Add onions, green pepper, garlic, fresh basil, salt, and veggie chik seasoning. Stir for about one minute, and then add tomatoes and honey. Sprinkle in the flour and blend in.

Place Brussels sprouts in a casserole dish, and cover with sauce.

Creamy Spinach with Rice Cheese

1 ½ lbs. fresh spinach leaves
2 cups water
¼ cup onions, chopped
1 tsp salt to taste
1 tbsp olive oil
2 tsp arrowroot
2/3 cups coconut milk
1 tbsp fresh lemon juice
¼ cup rice cheese, shredded

Wash fresh spinach thoroughly, in several changes of cold water to remove all the grit. Break spinach in 2–3 inch pieces.

Pour two cups water in medium size pot, add spinach and green onions, cook for 3 minutes. Add salt and olive oil. Stir in to blend, and cook for 3–4 minutes more. Drain liquid from spinach.

Place in sauce pan coconut milk, salt, olive oil and arrowroot. Blend until smooth, then add lemon juice and blend again. Cook sauce over medium, and stir until it begins to thicken.

Place spinach in a casserole dish and top with creamy sauce. Sprinkle top with soy baco bits.

Note: This dish goes well with rice.

Place in sauce pan coconut milk, salt, olive oil and arrowroot. Blend until smooth, then add lemon juice and blend again.

Place over medium heat in sauce pan and stir until it begins to thicken. Add rice cheese and blend in.

Herb Roasted Vegetables

3 cups cauliflower, broken off into florets
2 cups brussels sprouts, cut in half
2 medium carrots, cut into sticks
1 medium yam, cut in medium size slices
3 tbsp garlic, minced
1 tbsp olive oil
1 tbsp fresh rosemary, chopped
2 tsp fresh thyme, chopped
2 tsp fresh parsley, chopped
2 tsp lemon juice
1 tsp sea salt

Preheat oven to 450 degrees.

Place all ingredients in a large bowl. Toss vegetables to blend. Place vegetables in casserole dish. Roast for 20 minutes, turn vegetables over. Increase temperature to 500 degrees and roast vegetables 10 minutes more, or until tender. While roasting, the vegetables should be turned over 2–3 times.

Honey Carrots

6–8 medium carrots
3 cups water
1 tsp sea salt
2 tbsp cornstarch or arrowroot
1 tbsp lemon juice
¼ cup coconut milk
¼ cup honey or rice syrup
¼ cup coriander or cinnamon

Peel and cut carrots into 1-inch chunks. Place water in pot, and add salt. Let it come to a boil. Add carrots, then lower heat. Cook until carrots are folk tender.

Place corn starch into a small bowl, add lemon juice, coconut, honey and coriander. Blend until smooth. Pour over carrots in the pot. Stir until mixture thickens, stirring occasionally.

Note: If there is too much liquid in the pot after the carrots have cooked, pour some of the liquid off before adding thickener and save in case you need to add it back again.

Mock Cottage Cheese Loaf

14 oz. firm tofu
2 onions, chopped fine
4 cloves garlic, minced
2 stalks celery, chopped fine
1 bell pepper, chopped fine
1 cup of sour cream
½ cup mushrooms, finely chopped
¼ cup fresh lemon juice
1 cup walnuts, finely chopped
1 tsp sage
1 tsp poultry seasoning
1 tbsp veggie beef seasoning
2 cups wheat bread crumbs

Place mixture in loaf pan and cover with foil. Bake at 350 degrees for 1 hour.

Slice and serve with brown gravy.

Pecan Loaf

1 cup pecan meal
½ cup red bell peppers, chopped
1 onion, chopped
2 cups block rice cheese, grated
14 oz. firm tofu
1 cup whole wheat bread crumbs
1 tbsp Spike seasoning
2 tsp poultry seasoning
1 tsp sea salt

Mix all ingredients and place in a loaf pan. Cover with foil and bake at 350 degrees for one hour.

Vegetables and Entrée Dishes

Sugar Peas with Carrots

3 cups sugar peas, remove strings and steams
4 baby carrots, chopped (3 inch length) and steamed
2 tbsp olive oil
¼ cup onions, chopped
2 tsp sesame oil
¼ cup cashew nuts, chopped
½ cup water
1 tbsp veggie chik seasoning
1 tsp Celtic Sea Salt®

Heat oil in sauce pan over medium low heat. Add onion and sauté 2 minutes, or until soft.

Place in blender, cashew nuts, water, veggie chik seasoning and salt,
Add to sauce pan until it thickens.

Put sugar peas and carrots into a dish and top it with sauce.

Tasty Greens

1 bunch of fresh mustard greens, cut into bite size pieces
1 bunch of fresh turnips, cut in bite size pieces
1 bunch collards, cut into bite size pieces
6 cups water
1 small onion, chopped
1 tbsp nutritional yeast
3 lg cloves garlic, minced
2 tbsp honey
1 tsp sea salt
2 tbsp olive oil
1 tbsp veggie chik seasoning
¼ cup soy baco bits

Pour 6 cups of water into a large pot. Let the water come to a boil, then add onion, garlic, honey, salt, olive oil and veggie chik. Reduce the heat and let seasoning cook for three minutes.

Add the greens and cover the pot with a top. Lower the heat more and cook for thirty five minutes, or until tender.

Note: Add more seasoning for taste if needed.

Note: This recipe is a tasty meal with cornbread, and yams.

Delightful Pasta Dishes

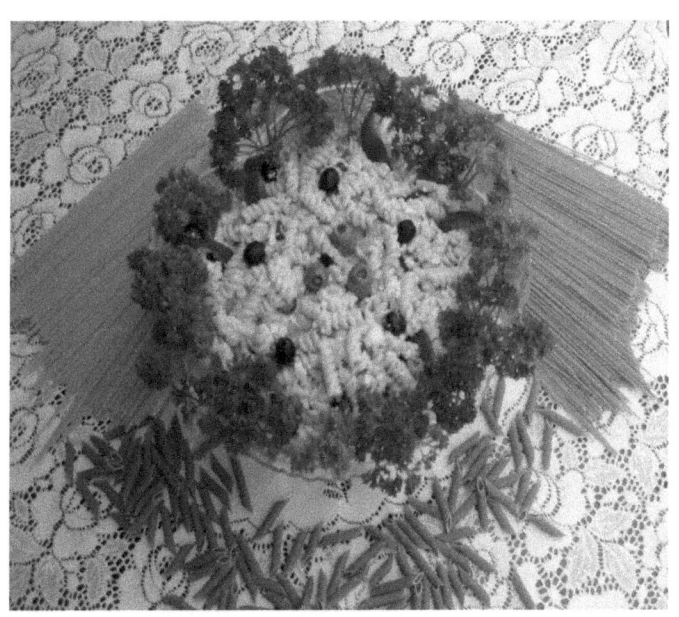

Artichoke Pesto Pasta

8 oz. artichoke pasta, boiled and drained
½ cup medium onion, chopped
⅓ cup parsley, minced
¼ cup pine nuts or walnuts, chopped
2 cloves garlic, minced
2 tbsp olive oil
¼ lb. extra firm tofu, mashed
4 oz. artichoke hearts, drained and chopped
½ cup green olives, sliced
1 fresh lemon juice
1 tbsp fresh basil, minced
½ tsp cayenne pepper
1 tsp sea salt

Pour oil in skillet, add tofu, garlic, onion, salt and cayenne. And cook over low heat. Cook while stirring for 3 minutes.

In a serving bowl, add parsley, basil, pine nuts, artichoke hearts and olives with cooked pasta. Cut lemon in half and sprinkle over pasta. Mix in sauté vegetables and tofu and toss to blend.

Curried Penne

8 oz. whole wheat penne pasta, boiled and drained
3 tbsp almonds, slivered
1 tbsp olive oil
½ onion, finely chopped
1 roma tomato, diced and crushed
1 ½ tsp curry
1 cup frozen tiny peas
¼ cup yellow bell peppers
½ tsp cumin
2 tbsp fresh cilantro, chopped
1 tsp salt
8 oz. coconut milk

Heat almonds over medium heat in skillet and stir 2–3 minutes until lightly brown. Add oil, tomato, cumin, curry, cilantro, yellow peppers, peas and salt. Cook 2–3 minutes while stirring. Add coconut milk and blend.

Cover skillet and let simmer 3 minutes. Pour mixture over pasta and blend.

Home Made Spaghetti with Sauce

8 oz. wheat spaghetti, boiled
½ cup textured vegetable protein flakes or granules, soak in warm water
2 tbsp olive oil
¾ cup onions, chopped
¼ cup celery, chopped
¼ cup bell peppers, chopped
3 cloves garlic, minced
¼ cup mushrooms, chopped
2 tbsp fresh basil, chopped
1 tbsp fresh oregano leaves, minced
1 tsp sea salt
1 tbsp spike seasoning
3 large roma tomatoes, diced and crushed
8 oz. tomato sauce
6 oz. tomato paste
1 tbsp honey

Pour oil in medium size skillet and place over medium heat. Add onion, celery, bell pepper, garlic, mushrooms, basil and oregano. Sauté for two minutes. Add roma tomatoes, tomato sauce, tomato paste and honey. Stir 1 minute to blend. Cover skillet with top and simmer on low for 15 minutes.

Serve spaghetti and top with sauce and vegan cheese.

Delightful Pasta Dishes

Meatless Lasagna

½ package of durum wheat lasagna
2 tbsp olive oil
½ cup onions, chopped
½ cup celery, chopped
½ cup red bell peppers, chopped
4 cloves garlic, chopped
3 tomatoes, chopped in small pieces
½ cup tomato paste
2 tbsp fresh basil, minced
2 tbsp honey
1 tsp salt to taste
2 tsp nutritional yeast (optional)
1 lb. block rice cheese, shredded (or sliced cheese)

Pour olive oil in skillet and place medium low heat. Add onions, celery, bell peppers and garlic. Sauté vegetables 2–3 minutes while stirring. Add tomatoes, basil, honey, salt and nutritional yeast. Crush the tomatoes and stir to blend in. Cover skillet and let simmer for five minutes.

Layer dry lasagna in casserole dish with sauce, next cheese, then sauce again. With the top layer should end up with sauce and cheese on the top. Cover with foil and bake at 350 degrees for 30 minutes or until done.

Pasta and Chard

5 oz. shell macaroni, boiled
3 cups of fresh chard, chopped
⅓ cup water
1 tbsp veggie chik seasoning
1 tbsp olive oil
¼ cup onions, chopped
2 cloves garlic, minced
8 oz. coconut milk
1 tbsp honey
4 oz. rice cheese, shredded
1 tsp sea salt

Rinse chard in cold water several times, chop and add to a medium size pot with oil and water. Add onions, garlic, chard and salt. Stir for five minutes, or until chard is tender. Add coconut milk and honey. Stir to blend. Next add rice cheese.

Wheat Noodles with Walnuts

10 oz. whole wheat durum semolina
3 cups broccoli, cut into small florets
1 cup small red bell peppers, chopped
2 tbsp toasted walnut, or olive oil
1 12 oz. pkg. extra-firm tofu, drained and cubed
2 cloves garlic, minced
¼ cup walnuts, chopped (or almonds, slivered)
1 tbsp maple syrup
1 cup fresh pomegranate seeds
5 green onions, chopped
1 tsp sea salt, chik seasoning and nutritional yeast

1. Add pasta and a pinch of salt to boiling water. Cook for 9 minutes.
2. Drain off water from noodles and set aside. 3. Heat 1 tbsp oil in skillet over medium heat.
4. Add tofu cubes to skillet, and sprinkle with sea salt, chik seasoning and nutritional yeast.
5. Cook for 10 minutes or until brown.
6. Remove from heat, add garlic and stir for 30 seconds until fragrant. Stir in walnuts, maple syrup and remaining walnut oil, or olive oil.
7. Toss pasta mixture with tofu mixture, pomegranate seeds and green onions.

Satisfying Rice Dishes

Brown Rice with Cranberries

1 cup long grain brown rice, steamed
½ cup dried cranberries
1 cup water
1 tbsp veggie chik seasoning
2 tbsp maple syrup
1 tbsp olive oil
¼ cup celery, finely chopped
2 tbsp green onions, chopped
½ cup mushrooms, sliced (optional)
2 tsp poultry seasoning
¼ cup fresh parsley, chopped
1 tsp sea salt
⅓ cup toasted pecans, chopped

Pour into blender, water, veggie chik seasoning, maple syrup, olive oil, poultry seasoning and salt. Blend 1 minute. Place in medium skillet. Add celery, green onions, parsley, mushrooms and cranberries. Cover skillet and simmer 3 minutes. Add brown rice and blend in roasted pecans.

Preheat oven to 350 degrees. Place pecans on cookie sheet and bake five minutes. Do not over bake.

Spanish Brown Rice

1 cup long grain rice
2 tbsp olive oil
2 cups water, warmed
½ cup tomato paste
2 cups roma tomatoes, chopped
1 tbsp honey
¼ cup celery, chopped
1 small yellow onion, chopped
3 cloves garlic, minced
½ bell pepper, chopped
1 small Serrano chili pepper, seeded and minced
2 tsp cumin
1 tsp sea salt
1 tbsp veggie chik seasoning, (optional)

Place rice in skillet with oil, over low heat. Stir and brown the rice for two minutes. Slowly add warm water. Cover skillet and cook rice on slow for twenty minutes or until done.

Add all other ingredients and stir. Cover skillet and place heat on very low. Simmer for 10 minutes.

Tofu Fry with Potatoes and Rice

3 cups long grain brown rice, cooked
2 tbsp olive oil
½ small onion, chopped
3 cloves garlic, minced
¼ cup red bell peppers, chopped
1 cup potatoes, diced
1 tsp sea salt
4 oz. tofu crumbled
⅓ cup water
¼ cup organic vegan ketchup

Pour olive oil and water into a medium size skillet. Add all vegetables and sauté for 3 minutes or until done. Add tofu and ketchup and continue to cook for 3 minutes. Blend in rice.

Vegetable Style Brown Rice

1 cup long grain brown rice
½ cup onions, chopped
2 cups zucchini, chopped
3 cloves garlic, minced
1 tbsp olive oil
½ cup green peppers, chopped
2 large tomatoes, chopped
2 ¾ cups water
1 tbsp veggie chik seasoning
1 tsp Celtic Sea Salt®

Put into a small casserole dish, brown rice, water salt, olive oil and veggie chik seasoning. Bake rice for 35 minutes, or until almost done. Remove rice from oven and add vegetables, toss together. Cover dish and place back in oven. Bake 10 minutes more, or until done.

Wild Rice Fiesta with Lentils and Tortilla Strips

4 cups French lentils, cooked and drain (set aside and save liquid)
2 tbsp olive oil
2 cups wild rice, steamed
1 yellow onion, chopped
4 cloves garlic, minced
1 4 chipotle chilies, seed and chopped
⅓ cup soy baco flakes (optional)
2 tbsp veggie chik seasoning
2 sweet potatoes or yams, cubed in small pieces
4 small corn tortillas, cut into thin strips
8 tbsp vegan sour cream
2 green onions, chopped
1 tbsp fresh cilantro
1 tsp Celtic Sea Salt®

Heat oil in large pot over low heat, add onion, garlic and chipotle chilies. Sauté for 3–4 minutes over low heat. Add liquid from cooked lentils and sweet potatoes. Cover with top and simmer for 20 minutes, or until potatoes are tender. Add soy baco flakes, veggie chik seasoning and salt.

Cook tortilla strips in small skillet, over medium heat for 3–5 minutes, or until crispy on both sides.

Ladle rice and lentil mixture in bowls and top each with soy cream, green onion and strips of tortilla.

Satisfying Rice Dishes

Wild Rice Pilaf with Vegetables

¾ cup long grain brown rice, uncooked
¼ cup wild rice, uncooked
3 cups water
2 tbsp veggie beef seasoning
1 tsp sea salt
1 green onion, finely chopped
3 cloves garlic, minced
2 stalks celery, chopped
1 tbsp honey
½ tsp ground clove
¼ cup pecans

Pour into medium sauce pot, 3 cups water, add veggie beef seasonings and sea salt. Bring to a boil. Add rice and then put heat on low. Cover pot and simmer rice for 40 minutes, or until tender. Add all other ingredients, blend gently with rice. Cover, and cook for 10 minutes more.

Brown pecans lightly in a skillet remove and blend with rice and vegetables.

Wild Rice with Butternut

3 cup wild rice, steamed
1 lb. butternut squash, peeled, seeded, and diced in small cubes
2 tbsp olive oil
1 medium fennel bulb, finely chopped
1 cup onions, chopped
3 cloves garlic, chopped
½ cup red bell peppers, chopped
1 tbsp fresh oregano, minced
1 tsp ground cumin
1 tsp salt
1 tbsp veggie chik seasoning
2 tsp nutritional yeast (optional)
⅓ cup water

Steam butternut and fennel in skillet with oil and water over low heat. Cover top and cook for 3 minutes. Add onion, garlic and red pepper. Stir to blend vegetables.
Add oregano, cumin, salt, veggie chick and nutritional seasoning, blend ingredient together with seasoning. Cover top and simmer on low 2–3 minutes.

Breads and Crackers

Amaranth Cereal

¼ cup amaranth cereal
⅛ tsp salt
1 cup water
¼ cup fresh blueberries
1 tbsp agave nectar or honey
dash of coriander or cinnamon
2 tsp olive oil (optional)

Place amaranth cereal in sauce pot with water and salt. Bring to a boil, then reduce heat and simmer for twenty minutes.

For taste add agaves nectar, drizzle with olive oil and sprinkle with coriander or cinnamon.

Basic Whole Wheat Bread

3 cups warm water
2 packages of active dry yeast
⅓ cup honey
5 cups unbleached bread flour
3 tbsp virgin olive oil
2 tsp Celtic Sea Salt®
3 ½ cups pastry wheat flour

Mix in a large bowl, warm water, yeast and ⅓ cup honey. Stir to blend, and then set aside until yeast has dissolved. Next add olive oil and salt and then blend in bread flour

Next stir in two cups of pastry wheat flour. Flour a flat surface and knead with pastry wheat flour until it is not real sticky. If it is still sticky to the touch, may add remaining pastry wheat flour, as needed. Form into ball and kneed.

Place into a greased bowl, turning once to coat the surface of the dough. Cover with a dish towel. Let rise in a warm place until doubled.

Punch down and divided into 3 loaves. Place in greased loaf pan and allow to rise until dough has topped the pans by one inch.

Bake at 350 degrees for 25–30 minutes. Lightly spray the tops with olive oil, to keep a hard crust from forming.

Fruity Nutty Granola

7 cups rolled oats
1 cup bran
1 cup sunflower seeds, raw
½ cup sesame seeds, unshelled
1 cup almonds, slivered
2 cups coconut, shredded, unsweetened
1 cup water
½ cup cashews or raw brazil nuts
1 cups dates, pitted
¼ cup dried papaya
¼ cup dried pineapple
1 ½ cup raisins
12 oz. fresh pineapple juice
2 tsp vanilla extract
1 tsp almond extract
1 tsp lemon extract
1 tsp coriander
½ tsp Celtic Sea Salt®

Mix in a large mixing bowl, oats bran, sunflower seeds, sesame seeds, almonds and coconut. In another bowl, water, cashews, dates, papaya, pineapple, raisins, pineapple juice, vanilla, almond extract, lemon extract, coriander and sea salt.

Combine the wet ingredients with the dry ingredients and mix well. Spread granola onto 2 or 3 baking sheets. Bake overnight, from 7–8 hours in oven at 170 degrees. Granola should be nice and crunchy. Sprinkle raisins and combine with granola when it is cool.

Note: For a healthier granola, combine all of the ingredients except the raisins, seeds, nuts and raisins. They contain heart healthy nutrients that will retain their antioxidants better when heat is not applied. After the granola has cooled, blend in the raisins, seeds, nuts and raisins. The granola will stay fresher when stored in the refrigerator.

Hardy Grain Cereal

1 cup long grain brown rice
1 cup millet
½ cup pearl barley
½ cup whole oats, (goats)
¼ cup red rice or wild rice
1 tsp Celtic Sea Salt® or Bragg Liquid Aminos
2–3 tsp nutritional yeast (optional)
herbal seasonings of your choice

Mix grains together and rinse in a small screened sieve. Place cereal in a thick bottom pot, add enough water, about two inches over the cereal. Add salt and blend in. Bring water to a boil, then turn down low, uncovered, cook about thirty five minutes or until done. If there is excess water, pour off.

This recipe will make a large amount and can be easily stored and used throughout the week. Recipe may be cut in back.

Cereal may be used the traditional way by using honey, another natural sweetener, and some soy, or rice milk.

Oatmeal Apple Pancakes

¾ cup pastry wheat flour
⅛ cup oats
2 tbsp Oat bran
½ tsp coriander or cinnamon
3 tsp non-aluminum baking powder
¼ tsp Celtic Sea Salt®
¼ cup raisins
½ cup apples, chopped
1 cup fresh apple juice
¼ cup silky tofu

Whisk all dry ingredients. Place in blender or vita mix, raisins, ½ cup apple, 1 cup fresh apple juice and silky tofu. Blend on low speed until liquefied. Add all dry ingredients and continue to blend until smooth. Pour batter by ¼ cupfuls on a nonstick skillet or griddle. Brown on both sides.

May be topped with stewed apples, honey, or maple syrup.

Pastry Wheat Raisin Nut Pancakes

2 cups pastry wheat flour
1 tsp sea salt
2 cups soy milk
2 tbsp honey
1 tbsp baking powder (non-aluminum)
¼ cup raisins
¼ walnuts, finely chopped

Combine flour and salt together. Mix together with a wire whisk.
Add to a blender two cups of soy milk and honey. Blend for 2–3 seconds. Add dry mixture to liquid and blend until smooth.

Pour mixture into a bowl and fold in raisins and walnuts. Brown on both sides in a non stick skillet.

Good with maple syrup, apple sauce, or your favorite topping.

Sun Seed Crackers

1 cup unbleached flour
¾ cup whole wheat flour
½ tsp non-aluminum baking powder
¼ tsp Celtic Sea Salt®
¼ cup sunflower seeds, crushed
2 tbsp onion, finely chopped
¼ cup soy mayonnaise
¼ cup soy yogurt
1 tbsp honey

Place in a medium mixing bowl, flour, baking powder salt and ground sunflower seeds. Stir together soy mayonnaise, soy yogurt and honey. Stir mayonnaise mixture into flour mixture till coarse crumbs form. Knead in bowl if necessary to mix.

Divide dough into 3 equal pieces. Roll each piece of dough out on parchment paper, or lightly floured surface. Roll dough out into about $1/16$ inch circle. Use a round cookie cutter to slightly score for each cracker. Prick the top with a fork. Remaining dough stripping from the circle, can be reformed into a dough ball and used to make more crackers.

Bake in a 350 degrees oven for 10–12 minutes or till lightly brown. Remove to a small rack to cool. Break apart each cracker.

Wholesome Grain Crackers

3 cups of pastry wheat flour
3 cups unbleached flour
½ cup sesame seeds
½ cup flax seeds
1 tbsp Celtic Sea Salt®
1 ⅜ cup olive oil
2 ⅛ cup warm water

Place flour, sesame seeds, flax seeds and salt in a large bowl. Blend this dry mixture with a wire whisk.

Pour oil and water together in one container and pour oil and water slowly into the flour mixture, stir while blending. If dough is too sticky, add a little more pastry wheat flour.

Mold dough together with hands and then separate the dough into three balls. Roll each dough ball out to ⅛ of an inch thickness, on a lightly floured surface or parchment paper. Place dough on cookie sheets and use a pizza cutter or knife to score it into 1 inch squares, or larger if desired. Bake at 350 degrees for 10 minutes, or until the edges began to turn brown.

Enjoy with salsa, dips, soups, peanut butter, or soy cream cheese.

Recipe may be cut in half to bake a smaller amount. Crackers will store well in freezer.

Guiltless Desserts

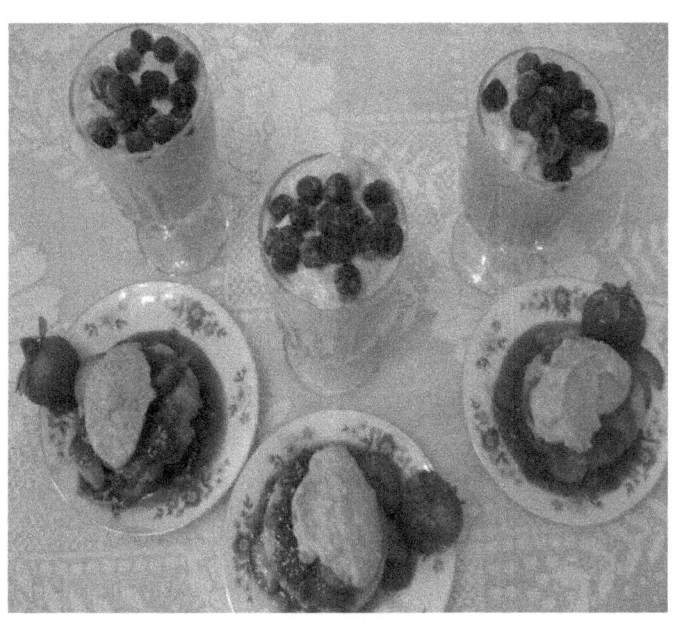

Apple Cake

1 ½ cup Fuji apples, chopped
½ cup sucanat or honey
¼ cup light virgin olive oil
⅓ cup walnuts, chopped
¼ cup raisins
1 tsp vanilla
⅓ cup silky tofu
1 cup pastry wheat flour
1 tsp non-aluminum baking powder
½ tsp coriander
¼ tsp sea salt

Place apples in a vita mix or food processor and blend apples into a sauce. Mix olive oil, sucanat, apple sauce, tofu and vanilla together. Mix well.

In a large bowl, combine pastry wheat flour, baking powder coriander and salt together, mix well. From food processor, add dry ingredients, mix well and then fold in walnuts and raisins. Bake at 350 degrees for 45 minutes.

Apple cake may be eaten plain, or with a topping, such as a fruit glaze.

Apricot Cake

2 cup dried apricots, chopped
1 ½ cups coconut, shredded
1 cup soya milk
1 cup pastry wheat flour
½ cup unbleached flour
2 tsp non-aluminum baking powder
¼ cup raisins (optional)
¼ cup pecans, chopped

Combine all ingredients, except the raisins and pecans in a bowl and mix well. Fold in the raisins and pecans.

Pour into a sprayed cake tin and bake at 350 degrees for 35 minutes, or until done. Test the center with a tooth pick. If it comes out dry, it is done.

Banana Cream Pie

1 vegan pie crust
½ cup sucanat
5 tbsp arrowroot
2 cups soy milk
½ tsp salt
1 tsp vanilla extract
2 ripe bananas
½ lb. firm tofu
2 tbsp almonds, coarsely chopped

Prepare pie crust according to directions

Combine sucanat and arrowroot together in a sauce pan and stir in soy milk and salt. Cook on low medium heat while stirring constantly until mixture becomes very thick. Remove from heat and stir in vanilla.

Drain tofu and blend it in a food processor until it is completely smooth. Add the pudding mixture and blend until smooth.

Slice the banana into thin rounds over the cool pie crust. Spread the tofu mixture on top.

Toast the chopped almonds in an oven at 375 degrees for 7–10 minutes, or until lightly brown. Sprinkle evenly over the pie. Refrigerate for at least 2 hours.

Carrot Cake

2 cups carrots, grated and cooked
1 cup raisins
1 ½ cups water
1 ½ tsp coriander
1 ½ tsp cinnamon
½ honey
½ tsp sea salt
½ cup unbleached flour
½ cup pastry wheat flour
2 tsp non-aluminum baking powder
¾ cup soy milk

Simmer the grated carrot, raisins, water and spices in a sauce pan for 10 minutes. Stir in honey and salt. Simmer for 2 minutes. Cool completely. Preheat oven to 250 degrees. In a large bowl, place the flour and baking powder, blend. Add the cooked carrots and soy milk with the rest of the mixture, blend well.

Spray a 9 inch pan with olive oil spray and fill with mixture. Bake at 350 degrees for 1 hour. Insert a tooth pick into center. It should come out clean to let you know it is ready.

Fruit Squares

Crumb Mixture

1 ½ cups whole wheat pastry flour
1 ½ cup rolled quick oats
1 tsp sea salt
½ cup fresh pineapple juice
½ cup unsweetened coconut, shredded

Place all ingredients together in a bowl, except for pineapple juice. Place in food processor and pulse about 5 times, for good mixture. Next pour pineapple juice slowly to mixture, just enough to moisture to hold dry ingredient together.

Filling

¼ cup sesame seeds
4 cups dates, chopped
¾ cup water
2 tbsp Eden® Agar flakes or arrow root powder
¼ cup honey (optional)
2 cups fresh pineapple, cubed
1 tsp vanilla
¼ cup nuts (walnuts, almonds or brazil nuts)

Place water and Eden® Agar flakes in sauce pan to soak for 10 minutes. Cook
On low heat while turning until it begins to thickens. Add honey and vanilla and blend. Combine with pineapple, sesame seeds and dates.

Pat half of crumb mixture into sprayed pyrex pan (9x12). Cover with date mixture, then rest of crumb mixture. Pat down well. Bake 30 minutes at 350 degrees. Let cool and break into squares.

Frozen Fruit Dessert

6 cups fresh peaches, frozen
8 pitted dates
3 cups fresh blue berries, frozen
3 bananas, frozen
8 oz. silky smooth tofu
⅓ cup honey

Wash and clean fresh peaches. Cut peaches into slices and place put on a cookie sheet, and freeze. Peel bananas, cut in slices and place in the freezer along with the blue berries. Freeze for several hours.

Combine the frozen fruit, dates, tofu and honey in a vita mix or electric blender. Blend on high speed until smooth and creamy.

Place frozen fruit in serving dishes. May garnish with granola and blueberries or raspberries.

Strawberry Biscuit Torte

⅓ cup extra virgin coconut oil (is natural bulk oil)
1 ¾ cups pastry wheat flour
2 ½ tsp non-aluminum baking powder
¾ tsp sea salt
¾ cup soy milk
1 lb. fresh strawberries, sliced

Heat oven to 450 degrees. Whisk together well flour, baking powder and salt. Cut the virgin coconut oil into the flour mixture. Pour in just enough milk, so dough will leave side of bowl. Too much will make it sticky, or not enough will make it dry.

Turn dough on lightly floured surface. Knead lightly 10 times. Roll ½ inch think, for making torte. Use a 3–4 inch biscuit cutter. Place on ungreased cookie sheet, about 1 inch apart. Bake to golden brown for 10–12 minutes. Split biscuits in half and top with fresh slice strawberries (glazed) and almond cream.

Strawberry Glaze

½ cup honey
½ cup fresh strawberries, crushed
½ tsp agar powder (or ½ tbsp agar flakes)
1 tsp coconut butter
½ tsp salt

Place all ingredients in sauce pan. Bring to a full boil, reduce heat and simmer for three minutes, stirring occasionally. Set aside to set.
Fold in fresh strawberries with glaze.

Almond Date Nut Cream

1 cup raw almonds (soaked for several hours)
1 cup water
1 cup dates

Blend all ingredients until smooth

The Whole Apple Pie

6 large fugi apples
8 oz. apple juice concentrate
4 oz. coconut cream
¼ cup honey (optional)
2 tbsp pastry wheat flour
2 tsp coriander seasoning
1 tsp vanilla
1 tsp salt

Core apples, but do not peel. Slice apples in ¼ inch slices. Place in blender apple concentrate juice, coconut cream, honey, vanilla and salt. Blend well.

Pour mixture in sauce pot and simmer for 5 minutes, or until it lightly thickens. Place apple slices on top of bottom pie crust and cover with sauce mixture, next cover with a top crust and flute edges. Bake 350 degrees for 30 minutes or until crust is brown.

Two Pie Crust

3 cups pastry wheat flour
1 tsp salt
1 cup virgin coconut oil (natural bulk, concentrated oil)
14 tbsp ice water

Pulse flour and salt in food processor several times to combine.
Add coconut concentrated oil and pulse 5 or more times until mixture resembles coarse sand.

Add water into mixture in food processor. Pulse until dough comes together.
Divide dough and roll into two balls. Roll dough out on two large pieces of wax paper. Press dough into two pie plate dishes. Slip dishes into plastic bags, tie in and chill for one hour. Use both pie crusts for top and bottom of one pie.

Tropical Fruitcake

3 tbsp active dry yeast
½ cup warm apple juice
⅓ cup honey
¼ cup applesauce
8 oz. apple juice
½ cup coconut cream
½ cup whole wheat pastry flour
1 ½ cups unbleached flour
1 tsp sea salt
½ cup dates
½ cup dried apricots
½ cup dried papaya
½ cup dried pineapple
1 tbsp fresh lemon juice
½ cup brazil nuts
½ cup black walnuts

Place yeast in large bowl, soften yeast in warm apple juice. Add honey, apple sauce and apple juice. Add coconut cream to mixture. Mix flour and salt together and blend with mixture in bowl. Mix dried fruits, nuts and lemon juice, blend thoroughly with batter.

Place in cake pans or miniature bread pans up to ¾ inches from top. Place loaf pans in a warm place. When raised to the top of pans, place in oven and bake at 350 degrees for 1 hour, then turn heat down to 325 degrees for the last 15 minutes, if it has browned sufficiently.

Yammy Pecan Mini Tarts

Filling

2 tbsp Eden® Agar flakes or arrow root powder
1 ½ cup soy milk
⅓ cup pure maple syrup
2 cups sweet potatoes or yams, cooked and mashed
1 tsp sea salt
½ tsp coriander, ground
1 tsp cardamom

To prepare filling, place agar flakes and soy milk in a bowl to soak for 10 minutes. Place mixture in a sauce pan and add maple syrup. Bring to a boil. Lower heat and simmer 15 minutes while stirring until flakes melts. Place in a blender and add sweet potatoes, salt, coriander and cardamom to blend.

Crust

2 cups pastry wheat flour
¼ tsp sea salt
½ tsp non-aluminum baking powder
¼ cup extra virgin coconut oil (is a natural bulk oil)
½ cup soy milk
½ cup pecan halves

To prepare crust, mix dry ingredients in bowl. Blend coconut concentrate oil and milk in blender for 1 minute. Add to dry ingredients and form into a ball. Divide the dough into (12–14) 1 to 1 ½ inch balls. Place the dough balls into sections of a mini-muffin tin. Press thumb into each ball and shape dough into cups.

When all cups have been filled, place in the center of cup a pecan. Bake at 350 degrees for 20–25 minutes, until crust is golden brown.

Eating More Raw for a Healthier Life

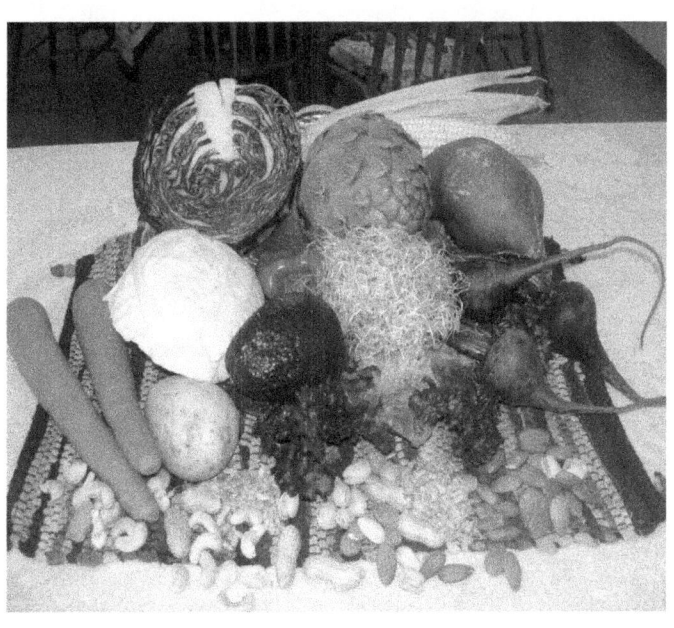

Carrot Latte Soup

1 ½ cups fresh carrot juice
1 cup fresh coconut milk
½ tsp jalapenos, seeded and minced
½ tsp fresh ginger, minced
½ tsp garlic, minced
⅓ cup avocado
2 tsp olive
1 tsp sea salt
1 tbsp fresh basil leaves, chopped

Blend all of the above ingredients and place into a serving bowl. Set aside.

For garnish, the following ingredients are suggested. Replace with other vegetable if desired.

2 tbsp avocado, diced
2 tsp mint leaves, chopped
2 tsp red bell peppers, diced
1 tsp scallions, chopped

Corn Chowder Soup

4 ears raw fresh sweet corn
½ large cucumber, diced
1 tbsp nutritional yeast (optional)
1 tsp sea salt
2 tsp fresh oregano (or dried)
2 tsp ground cumin
3 tsp fresh green onions, minced
¾ cup water

Choice of additional ingredients that can be added:

3 tsp Bragg Liquid Aminos
1 pinch of cayenne pepper
2 tsp veggie chik seasoning
2 tsp fresh pressed garlic juice
1 cup mixture of red bell peppers, celery and parsley

Cut the corn off the cobs. Set aside the kernels from one of the cobs. Place the remaining kernels into a blender and all the remaining ingredients. Blend until smooth. Add small amounts of water if needed. Pour soup puree into bowls. Stir in the extra vegetables and the corn that was set aside.

Fennel Salad Combo

½ head fennel, chopped finely
1 small head chicory
½ romaine lettuce (use lower part, cut from middle to end) shred finely
¼ cup basil leaves, chopped
10 cherry tomatoes, cut in halves
1 yellow apple, diced

Rosemary dressing

6 tbsp olive oil
2 tbsp apple cider vinegar (optional)
2 tbsp fresh lemon juice
1 tsp fresh rosemary, chopped
1 tbsp honey (optional)
2 tsp Bragg Liquid Amino or ½ tsp salt

Toss vegetables and apple well. Place in a serving bowl. Blend dressing and pour over top of salad. Toss and serve.

Gazpacho Power Soup

4 large tomatoes
½ cucumber
¼ cup red bell pepper, chopped
1 garlic clove
2 stalks celery
2 tsp Bragg Liquid Aminos (optional)
½ tsp sea salt

May be garnished with:

½ avocado, cubed
3 tsp fresh basil leaves, minced
3 tsp scallions, chopped

Blend or juice vegetables. Add to soup the following garnish. Other vegetables of your choice may replace the suggested vegetables if desired.

Green Life Soup

3-5 collard green leaves
3-5 kale leaves
¼ cup parsley, chopped
2 cloves garlic
⅓ cup red onion
2 cloves garlic
⅓ cup green onions, chopped
2 tbsp fresh lemons juice
1 avocado, remove skin and seed
2 yellow peppers
½ tsp sea salt
2 tsp chili powder (more to taste if desired)
¼ cup edamame beans, shelled
½ cup pumpkin seeds, ground
2 cups water

Combine 1 cup of water and edamame beans into a vita mix. Blend until smooth, add all other vegetables, one at a time. Add 1 cup of water and ground pumpkin seeds. Blend well.

This recipe has great nutritive value. It is filled with vitamins, calcium and minerals.

Healthy Creamy Coleslaw

½ small red cabbage, finely shredded
1 cup green cabbage, finely shredded
½ yellow onion, chopped
½ cucumber, diced
2 cups cashew nuts (or sunflower seeds if preferred)
1 cup fresh celery juice
2 tbsp fresh lemon juice
2 tbsp fresh parsley, chopped
1 cup fresh almond or soy milk
¼ cup edamame beans, shelled
1 tsp fresh thyme, minced
2 tsp fresh dill, minced
½ tsp salt

Place cabbage, onion and cucumber in a serving bowl and toss to blend.

Place in a vita mixer cashew nuts and blend into a fine meal. Add celery juice, lemon juice and fresh almond milk. Blend 1 minute. Add edamame beans and blend well to mix in. Add parsley, thyme and dill. Blend well. Pour dressing over vegetables in bowl and toss to mix in.

Life Thriving Soup

1 cucumber, with peeling, chopped
1 red pepper, chopped
2 stalks celery, chopped
3 roma tomatoes
¼ cup edamame beans, shell beans
3 tbsp fresh lemon juice
3 cloves garlic, chopped
½ red onion, chopped
2 tbsp cold pressed oil, or flax oil
1 bunch cilantro
2 tsp ginger root, minced
½ beet, chopped
1 ¼ cup ground sesame seeds, ground
¼ cup Bragg Liquid Amino (or 1 tsp of salt)
¼ tsp cayenne
2 tbsp chili powder
2 ½ cups water

Place all chopped vegetables into a vita mix. Add lemon juice, garlic, onion, cilantro, Bragg, cayenne, chili powder and water. Blend for about 45 seconds. Add ground sesame meal. Blend until smooth.

Mellon Soup

2 ½ cups watermelon, seeded and cubed
2 ½ cups cantaloupe, seeded and cubed
2 cups of mango, seeded and diced
¼ cup lime juice
3 tbsp fresh mint, chopped
1 tbsp fresh ginger, minced
1 tbsp honey
⅛ tsp ground cardamom
⅛ tsp Bragg Liquid Aminos (optional)

Put half the cubed watermelon and half the cubed cantaloupe and 1 cup of mango in a food processor and blend until smooth, combine the remaining cubed watermelon and cubed cantaloupe to the soup, add the mango.

Combine the lime juice, mint, ginger, honey, cardamom and Bragg Liquid Aminos. Add to the mixture and blend. Chill and serve.

Nutty Loaf

2 cups of sunflower seeds
½ cup pumpkin seeds
¼ cup brown sesame seeds, soaked over night
1 cup of almonds
¼ cup carrot, graded
⅓ cup potatoes, grated
¼ cup fresh baby green peas
1 tbsp fresh parsley, minced
¼ cup fresh yellow onions, diced small
1 tbsp Bragg Sprinkle Seasoning (or 1 tsp salt)

Mix well all ingredients, and with your hands, form the shape and put it in a loaf pan. If there is a dehydrator available, you may want to dehydrate the loaf for a dryer loaf.

Quinoa Veggie Mix

½ cup sprouted quinoa
½ cup roma tomatoes, chopped
⅓ cup edamame beans, shelled
2 tbsp Bragg Liquid Aminos
¼ cup fresh squeezed lemon juice
½ cup fresh onions, diced
¼ cup hiccama or burdock, diced
¼ cup cucumber, diced
1 cup fresh parsley
1 tbsp garlic, minced
1 tbsp jalapenos, seeded, veined and diced
2 tbsp ginger, diced
⅓ cup olive oil
1 tbsp honey (optional)

Combine all ingredients into a serving bowl. Mix well and serve.

Juicing for Life

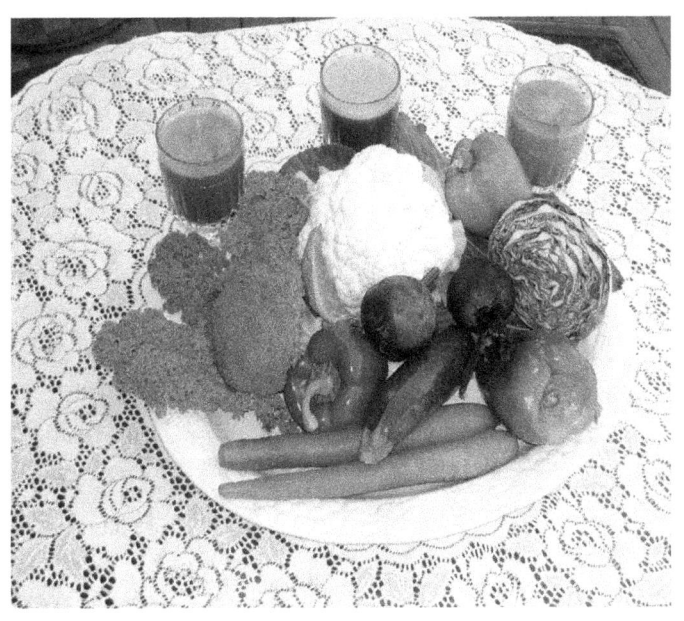

Brain Tonic Malt

1 cup blueberries
½ cup cranberries
1 small banana
1 cup fresh coconut milk
1 tbsp flax seed, ground
8 almond seeds, ground
2 tsp kelp

Flax seeds and almonds will grind together in a vita mix. Place all ingredients into vita mix and add coconut milk. If malt is too thick, more coconut milk can be added.

Cleansing Remedy

¼ small head cabbage, juiced
3 carrots, juiced
1 tbsp fresh ginger, chopped
2 cloves garlic
1 tsp Bragg Liquid Aminos (optional)

Place all ingredients in vita mix, blend and drink

Energy Boost Smoothie

1–2 large carrots, washed and juiced
1 celery stalk, with leaves, washed
1 small beet root, washed chopped and juiced
few leaves of parsley (equal to 1 cup packed parsley), washed and chopped
few leaves of watercress (equal to 1 cup packed watercress leaves), washed
few leaves of spinach (equal to 1 cup packed spinach leaves), washed
3 tomatoes, washed and steamed, cut in quarters
sea salt or other seasoning to taste

Place all ingredients in vita mix and blend. Drink right away.
***Use less leaves if drink is too bulky.

Green Smoothies

1 tbsp flax seeds
10 almonds
2 cups fresh carrot juice
1 large red apple, chopped
2 or more fresh collard green leaves (or more depending on size of leaf)
2 fresh kale leaves
2 fresh mustard green leaves, or swiss chard
½ cup fresh parsley, chopped

Place flax seeds and almonds in the vita mix and blend until the seeds and nuts are close to powdered. Add 2 cups of carrot juice and then blend.

Add apple and blend again. Add all the greens and blend till smooth.
Drink immediately, while the enzymes are fresh and alive.
Drink at least 3–4 days a week.

Note: kale, swiss chard, collards, beet, turnips and mustard greens are packed with vitamins, minerals, fiber and an array of photochemicals that may reduce heart disease risk, eye diseases and certain cancer.

Collards belong to the cabbage family, called cruciferae. It is known to be the richest in nutrient elements.

Mid-Day Boost

1 large red apple, chopped
4 asparagus (use tender parts only)
1 stalk celery, chopped
1 small tomato
⅓ cup cucumber, sliced
2 cups carrot juice

Combine all ingredients into a vita, and blend until smooth.

Nourishing Drink

3 cups of fresh carrot juice
1 cup parsley
1 small green apple, quartered
4 broccoli florets

Remove stem from apple and wash. Do not remove seeds, they are full of nutrients. Do not remove skins from carrots, scrub the skin while washing. Juice the carrots and pour in the carrot juice. Add all the other ingredients into a vita mix and blend well.

Peachy Cream

2 peaches, washed and pitted
¼ cup golden raisins
½ banana
1 cup coconut milk

Slice peaches in several pieces, place in blender and add other ingredients. Process until smooth.

Power House Fruit Smoothie

1 tbsp flax seeds, ground
10 almonds, ground
2 cups rice or soy milk
¼ cup raisins
⅓ cup blueberries
1 large red apple, stemmed and quartered
1 banana

Place flax seeds and almonds in vita mix. Add rice or soy milk, add apple and blend to smooth. Add all other ingredients and blend well.
This smoothie is so nourishing and filling, it's almost like a meal. Added to your breakfast, it will stay with you a good part of the day.

Springaide

3 large red apples, juiced
1 tbsp fresh lemon, squeezed
4 kiwis
2 tsp honey (optional)

Remove skin from kiwi, combine with other ingredients in vita mix and blend well.

Sprouting Life

1 handful of sunflower sprouts
½ cup bean sprouts
1–2 tsp spiraling powder (or spiraling flakes)
1 large apple
3 cups fresh carrot juice

Combine all ingredients into a vita mix and blend well.

Yammy Veggie

⅓ cup sweet potatoes
2 large tomatoes
1 large celery stalk
1 cup fresh carrot juice
1 clove garlic
¼ cup green pepper, chopped
¼ tsp fresh ginger

Scrub skin of potatoes and chop into pieces. Place potato pieces in vita mix and add the rest of the ingredients.

Dairy Alternatives

Coconut Butter

1 ¼ cup coconut oil, unrefined organic
¾ cup light olive oil
2 tbsp liquid lecithin
3 tbsp flax seed oil
1 cup water (distilled preferably)
1 tbsp Celtic Sea Salt®

If less oil is desired, add 1 cup cooked millet or quinoa.

Combine all ingredients into a blender or vita mix, except for cooked cereal, if desired. Blend until smooth, then add cooked cereal if you plan on using it.

The coconut butter may be used on toast, hot cereal, for baking and on potatoes or vegetables.

The coconut oil is an organic unrefined cold pressed extra virgin coconut oil. It has no trans or hydrogenated fat, no cholesterol or hexane, which is used to extract edible oils from seeds and vegetables . No refrigeration required, it is solid at room temperature and melts at 76 degrees.

Not all saturated fat is bad! Coconut oil is cholesterol free and contains medium-chain good fats with 50% Lauric acid, it is a healthy nutrient that supports the metabolism.

Cheesy Pimento Cashew Sauce

1 cup cashews
½ cup water
¼ cup of roasted red peppers (or use pimentos from a jar)
2 tsp lemon juice
2 tbsp onions, chopped
1 clove garlic, minced
2 tsp yeast flakes
1 tsp Celtic Sea Salt®
1 pinch cayenne red pepper

This recipe is good over steamed broccoli, pizza and baked potatoes.

Roast red bell pepper with skin, turning to both sides, until the skin is dark.
Place pepper inside of a paper bag and let it sweat for 10–15 minutes, remove pepper and remove the skin. Set aside.

Rinse cashews nuts and place in a mixer, add water and blend well. Add roasted red pepper and remaining ingredients. Blend until smooth.

Dairy Free Butter

¼ cup extra virgin olive
¼ tsp sea salt
1 tsp liquid lecithin

Combine all ingredients and place in a blender or food processor. Put mixture in a small container and freeze until solid.

Fruity Butter Spread

¾ cup dates
¼ soft dried apricots
1 orange
1 tsp vanilla
1 ½ tbsp fresh lemon juice

Combine all ingredients in a blender, and process till smooth.

This goes well with toast, pancakes, waffles or muffins.

Hummus Three in One

16 oz. garbanzo beans, rinsed and drained
1 lemon, juiced
1 tbsp fresh garlic, minced
1 tsp Celtic Sea Salt®
¼ cup cold water
½ cup sesame Tahini
⅛ cup chives or fresh green onions, chopped
1 tsp cumin
⅓ cup roasted red peppers, jarred
⅓ cup fresh cilantro leaves

Combine all ingredients into food processor or blender except the roasted red peppers and the fresh cilantro. Blend until smooth.

Divide the hummus up into three bowls.

Bowl #1 Plain hummus
Bowl #2 Add ⅓ cup roasted red peppers and blend.
Bowl # 3 Add ⅓ cup cilantro and blend.

All three variations may be served as dips or sandwich spread.

Italian Tomato Sauce

28 oz. fresh Italian tomatoes, diced
6 oz. tomato paste
1 medium yellow onion, chopped
¼ cup celery, minced
¼ cup olive oil
2 tbsp green bell peppers, minced
6 cloves garlic, minced
¼ cup fresh basil, minced
¼ cup oregano, minced
1 tsp Celtic Sea Salt®
1 tsp fresh rosemary, minced
1 tsp fresh thyme, minced
1 tbsp honey

Place tomatoes and tomato paste in food processor. Pulse to break up in small pieces.
Add to heavy sauce pot, olive oil and onion. Stir over medium heat, until the onion becomes translucent, then add celery, green peppers and garlic. Sauté for five minutes. Add tomato, paste, basil, oregano, rosemary, thyme, salt and honey to sauce pot. Cover pot, simmer on low 20 minutes. This sauce works well with lasagna, pasta, pizza and eggplant.

Jalapeno Tofu Cheese

¾ cup water
½ cup cashews
⅗ cup firm tofu
2 tbsp nutrition yeast flakes
1 ½ tbsp fresh lemon juice
½ jalapeno pepper, minced (seeded and veins remove)
⅓ cup pimentos
1 tsp Celtic Sea Salt®
2 tsp onion powder
¼ tsp garlic powder

Combine all ingredients in a blender and process until smooth. Place cheese in a container and refrigerate to chill. Cheese will become thicker.

Other milder peppers may be used, according to your choice.

Non-Dairy Cottage Cheese

1 lb. firm tofu
½ tub Tofutti® Better Than Cream Cheese
½ tsp Celtic Sea Salt®
1 tsp onion powder
2 tbsp fresh squeezed lemon juice

Crumble tofu into a medium bowl and set aside.

Blend the following ingredients together and add to the crumbled tofu.
Mix well. Chill and serve.

This recipe goes well with a fruit salad and toast.

Other ingredients may be added, such as chive, onion veggie chik seasoning.

Nut Milk Alternatives Variations

A basic recipe can be used for all nut milks. Nuts that can be used are pecans, almonds, walnuts, brazil nuts, sunflower seeds and more. All you will need for a set up is a blender and strainer. Fine mesh may be used for a strainer, or a cheese cloth. Nut milks are a part of the raw food diet. Although the material is strained out, it can still be used for as a thickener for stews, soups and baking. Whole grain foods have all the nutritional properties necessary to make good blood.
Quotation #301 of 500, *God's Nutritionist*, page 104

Ellen White was one hundred years ahead of her time; she recognized that a plant-based diet resulted in good blood. As a matter of fact, the liquid from young coconuts was used in lieu of blood transfusions during World War II. It is a living fluid, filled with enzymes.

Young coconut milk is delicious right from the coconut. In this drink, is pure ambrosia. Nut milks are a raw living food. It is a meal in itself, it can be drunk for breakfast, lunch, or dinner. It replaces the extra-thick milkshakes.

Olive Butter

¼ cups extra virgin olive oil
¼ tsp salt
1 large clove garlic

Blend olive oil, sea salt and garlic together in a mixer. Blend until smooth.
Place olive butter in a small container and freeze for about 4 hours or until solid. This olive oil butter can be used like regular sticks of butter. It can be cut off in small squares and placed on steamed vegetable or baked potatoes.

Nut Milks

Nut or Seed Milk

1 cup any nuts or seeds, soaked overnight and drained
3 cups filtered water
1 tbsp raw honey or 4 pitted dates
1 tsp Celtic Sea Salt® (optional)

Place in blender all ingredients and blend until smooth.

Almond Milk

1 cup almonds, soaked over night
4 cups water
1 banana
1 tbsp raw honey
1 cup dates
¼ tsp salt

Combine all ingredients into blender.
Start blender on slow first, as ingredients begin to combine. After a few seconds, switch to high speed and blend until smooth.

Rice Cheese Spread

8 oz. block or sliced vegan rice cheese
1 8 oz. vegan cream cheese
1 tbsp garlic, minced
1 pinch cayenne pepper
2 tsp fresh basil leaves, chopped
2 tbsp green onions, chopped
1 ¼ cup virgin olive oil

Place rice cheese, vegan cheese and olive oil into a food processer, process for about 10 seconds. Add remaining ingredients. Spread may be stored in refrigerator for one week. Serve at room temperature. This spread works well over pizza, pasta, baked potatoes and on breads.

Roasted Red Pepper Spread

17 oz. jar roasted red peppers, drained and chopped
1 8 oz. vegan cream cheese
3 tbsp onions, finely minced
1 clove garlic, minced
¼ cup healthy green olives, drained and chopped

Combine all ingredients and blend well.
This spread works well on french bread, sandwiches or crackers. Adding salad vegetables makes a wonderful delicious addition.

Spinach Dip Blend

12 oz. Tofutti® Better Than Cream Cheese
4 oz. fresh spinach, chopped
¼ cup fresh basil
2 cloves garlic, minced
⅓ jar of artichoke hearts, rinsed and drained
1 tbsp fresh lemon juice
⅛ tsp Celtic Sea Salt®
1 pinch of cayenne (optional)

Drain tofu and set aside. Wash leaves of fresh spinach well and blot with paper towel to dry, then chop. Add to food processor, better than cream cheese, spinach, basil, artichoke hearts, lemon juice and cayenne pepper. Pulse until ingredients are coarsely chopped. Refrigerate until ready to serve.

Thai Peanut Sauce

2/3 cups peanut butter
1 cup coconut milk
1 tbsp honey
¼ cup light soy sauce or brags amino
3 cloves garlic, minced
2 green onions, diced
2 tbsp sesame oil
1 tbsp fresh ginger, minced
½ tsp cayenne pepper
juice from two limes
2 tbsp sesame seeds
2 tbsp green onions, minced

Combine all ingredients into a sauce pan, over low heat, stir while cooking until sauce begins to thicken, or come to a desired consistency.

This sauce will be good over a rice bowl, pasta noodles with vegetables, and salads.

The Best Mayonnaise

3 tbsp fresh lemon juice
1 cup silky soy tofu
3 tbsp liquid lecithin
1 tbsp wheat germ oil
2 tbsp flax oil
2 tbsp soy protein powder
1 tbsp honey
½ tsp salt

Put all the ingredients in blender, except the lecithin, wheat germ oil and flax oil. Blend on the lowest speed, add oil one at a time and blend until it thickens and becomes smooth. Transfer to a jar.

See terms and definitions to define the ingredients in this recipe.

Homeward Bound Dietary Plan

Taking a journey and setting goals to have better health, may help to motive you to stay on track. Given a wide selection of foods to choose from, for breakfast, lunch and dinner, will help to make the decision easier for each meal.

The beauty of whole foods is that they are nutritionally packed, with fiber, protein, complex carbohydrates, natural fats and minerals. Dr. Hans Diel, DrHSc, mentions in his CHIP program, "Eat more, weigh less". The reason for that is, that wholesome food does it's job. It places itself where it needs to be. It does not stick around and plug up the system, or create illnesses.

Breakfast (Choose one type)

Cooked Grains
Brown (long or short grain)
Millet
Oats
Quinoa
Organic Yellow grits
Amaranth
Barley

Fresh Fruits (Choose two to three types for eating)

Apple
Pear
Grapes
Mango
Orange
Banana
Strawberries

Nuts and seeds

8-10 Raw Almonds
Raw Pumpkin seeds, Flax, or Sesame, sprinkle over cooked grains, put in a smoothie, or in recipe. Other nuts or seeds may also be used.

Breads (Choose 1 slice of bread or waffle)

Multigrain breads, or whole grain waffles, may be added to the breakfast meal.

Lunch (Choose one of each)

Salad Recipes (Check pages in book)
Green Bean Salad
Green Vegetable Salad
Potatoes Cucumber Salad
Black Bean Salad
Fruit Salad Mix
Cabbage Salad
Garbanzo Bean Salad
Kidney Bean Avocado Salad

Soup

Black French Lentil Soup
Northern Bean Soup
Tomato Tofu Soup
Creamy Broccoli Chowder Soup
Potatoes Vegetable Soup
Cream of Asparagus Soup
Cabbage Corn Chowder Soup
Black Bean Chili Soup

Breads

Homemade muffins, multigrain bread, or crackers may be eaten with the lunch meal. If buying from the market, look for a good healthy alternative, that has low sodium, no sugar and other healthy ingredients. Your health food store is your best bet.

Supper is the time to prepare your body for rest through the night. It must not be over loaded with heavy food. Supper should be light.

Supper

Popcorn
Fruit Salad
Bread
Crackers
Vegetable Soup

Fruit and Vegetable Combinations

Some have inquired about mixing vegetables and fruit together, and its possibilities of it causing indigestion. There are many cause of indigestion, including, stress, smoking, alcohol, ulcers and high fat diet. What many people do not realize, is that the most common forms of indigestion in basically healthy people can be prevented by simply eating the foods in the right combination. Or to avoid foods combinations that are likely to cause indigestion.

There are a number of different food groups, each group using a different enzyme or group of enzymes to digest that particular group.

People suffering from chronic indigestion, usually are mixing foods from groups that don't go together, because the enzyme that is required to digest each type of food, cancel each other out, therefore what happen is that the food ends up laying in your stomach for long periods of time.

What is important to understand, is that there are a number of food groups and each food group uses a different enzyme or group of enzymes to digest that particular group. Fruits should never be eaten with anything. If you are going to eat fruit, eat it as a snack by itself, or way after your meal is over as a dessert. Fruit will ferment with anything that you put with it.

The remaining food groups go well together. Protein and vegetables are excellent combinations. Digesting the right combination of foods each day will result in good nutrition for the building of your cells and tissue.

Herbal Seasonings

Aromatic Veggie Seasoning

¼ cup dried savory
¼ cup parsley
2 tbsp dried thyme leaves
1 tbsp sage
2 tbsp celery seeds
1 tbsp dried onion flakes
1 tsp dried lemon rind
1 tsp sea salt

Combine all ingredients in blender and whiz for 10–15 seconds.

Chili Powder

20 dried chilies
3 tbsp paprika
2 ½ tsp ground cumin
1 tsp dried parsley
1 tsp garlic powder
2 ½ tsp dried oregano
¼ tsp cayenne parsley
1 tsp sea salt or salt

Chili powder is a traditional blend of ground spices. It adds flavor to food and reduces the need for salt and other irritating spices.

Combine ingredients and mix well.

Curry Powder

1 tsp dried mustard
1 tbsp turmeric
2 tsp coriander
1 tsp each ground cumin and cayenne pepper
1 tsp cardamom
1 tsp ground ginger
1 tbsp fenugreek
½ tsp dried chili pepper
1 tbsp vegetarian chik seasoning

Italian Seasoning

2 tbsp dried basil
1 tbsp dried oregano
1 tbsp parsley
1 tsp sea salt
1 tsp rosemary, thyme, parsley and cayenne pepper

Combine all ingredients and mix well.

Savory Vegetable Seasoning

¼ cup dried savory
¼ cup dried parsley
2 tbsp dried thyme leaves
1 tbsp sage
2 tbsp celery seed
1 tbsp dried onion flakes
1 tsp dried lemon rind
1 tsp sea salt

Combine all ingredients in blender and process 10–15 seconds.

Veggie Chicken-Style Seasoning

4 tsp parsley flakes
4 tsp celery seeds
1 tsp turmeric
4 tsp onion flakes
¼ tsp savory seasoning
1 tsp sea salt
1 tsp organic cane juice

Combine all ingredients in blender and process 10–15 minutes

Herbal Seasonings for Vegetables, Fruit and Dressings

Beans	Sweet Basil, Oregano, Dill, Savory, Mint, Garlic, Bay Leaf, Parsley
Beets	Tarragon, Dill, Sweet Basil, Bay Leaf, Cardamom seeds, Lemon
Broccoli	Tarragon, Marjoram, Oregano
Cabbage	Caraway, Celery seed, Savory, Tarragon, Dill
Carrots	Sweet Basil, Dill, Marjoram, Thyme, Parsley
Cauliflower	Rosemary, Savory, Dill, Tarragon
Coleslaw	Dill, Marjoram, Caraway seeds, Savory, Mint
Eggplant	Sweet Basil; Thyme, Oregano, Sage
Fruit Salad	Mint, Rosemary, Lemon Balm
Green Beans	Sweet Basil, Parsley, Garlic, Marjoram, Rosemary, Thyme, Oregano, Savory
Green Salad	Sweet basil, Parsley, Garlic, Tarragon, Lemon, Thyme, Dill, **Dressing** — Marjoram, Oregano, Rosemary, Savory, Mint
Lima Beans	Sweet Basil, Garlic, Marjoram, Savory, Parsley
Potatoes	Dill, Garlic, Sweet Basil, Marjoram, Savory, Parsley
Peas	Sweet Basil, Mint, Savory, Oregano, Dill
Spinach	Tarragon, Thyme, Oregano, Rosemary
Squash	Sweet Basil, Dill, Oregano, Rosemary
Tomatoes	Sweet Basil, Parsley, Dill, Garlic, Savory

Terms, Definitions and Resources

Definition of Food Terms and Ingredients

Arrowroot Is a natural thickener that comes from the root of a tropical plant. It is high in minerals, not refined like cornstarch to thicken gravies, puddings, etc.

Eden® Agar Flakes Is a transparent seaweed, used to create an extract called Agar which is used by vegetarians as a substitute for gelatin.

Bragg Liquid Aminos Bragg Liquid Amino is a Certified non-GMO liquid protein concentrate derived from healthy soybeans, that contains 16 amino acids. Bragg Liquid Aminos has a small amount of naturally occurring sodium. No table salt is added. Bragg has no chemicals, no artificial coloring, no alcohol, no preservatives and no gluten. It is a source of delicious protein. It tastes good on salads, soups, beans, wok foods, tofu, dressings, gravies, potatoes, casseroles, veggies, etc. Yes, and even on popcorn.

Veggie Chik Is a unique blending of organic vegetables and herbs. The ingredients are soy flour, salt, food yeast, onion, garlic, parsley and celery. No black or white pepper, MSG, fat, dairy products or fillers. Broth or soup based, can be made by using 1 rounded tsp. of Veggie chik seasoning to 1 cup of hot water.

Tarragon Is an herb, grown inside or outside. It is a french herb. Tarragon is one of the spices included with chives, dill, and thyme, it may be added to soups, stews and other foods. Used fresh, the flavor is more intense. Use sparingly. Used dry the flavor is less tense.

Fenugreek Is a plant, its leaves and seeds are cultivated and used as a spice. It is great used in curry and flavoring. It has a rich source of carbohydrates, protein and vitamin A and C. It is perfect for curries and Indian dishes.

Turmeric Is a spice made from grinding the roots of the cumin plant. It is a prime ingredient for curry powder. It is used for condiments, rice dishes and sauces.

Marjoram Is a mint in the oregano family. It can be described as mild oregano. It works well with pasta, soups, beans, split pea or lentil soup. It enhances the flavor of most vegetables.

Mori-Nu Tofu Is made with non genetically (GMO) soy beans. It is velvety smooth. Silken style, perfect for everything, soups, smoothies, dips, cream pies and more.

Edamame	Are fresh baby soybeans that comes from the young pods, it is harvest before it hardens. They are quickly parboiled and frozen to retain their freshness. They carry lots of protein, calcium, vitamin A and they are high in fiber, phosphores and in photoestrogens, a natural plant estrogen.
Liquid lecithin	Is from soy. It health benefits are in choline and inosital. It is a pure vegetable product in its natural liquid state, it is not bleached. It may be used in shakes, cooked cereals, in sauces, salad dressings, gravies or baked goods, may be whipped into peanut butter, or making alternate butter. Lecithin is also non sticking. Mix two parts of it to one part of vegetable oil, or other oils. Brush on baking ware, just before baking or cooking in a skillet, or waffle irons.
Flax Oil	In flax oil is found a good source of omega-3. The organic vegetarian omega-3, comes from cold expell-pressed. It has a natural fresh taste. Flax particulate is the richest known plant source of lignan. Lignans are a group of plant nutrients called phytonutrients found in seeds.
Soy Organic Protein	Is a protein powder. It is vegan, all natural and is non GMO. It contains the highest quality of organic available. Unlike other soy proteins that use chemical extractions. This high quality vegan protein is rich in soy, is of lavones which promote hormonal and antioxidant balance.
Wheat Germ Oil	It is taken out of the germ from wheat. It can be used in breads, cereals, crackers, etc. It is a good source of fatty acid and is vital for the, growth of the body. It has exceptional nourishing qualities. It improves the circulation of blood in the skin, repairs skin cells, scar tissue and is good for stretch marks.
Bulgur Wheat	Is a quick form of whole wheat that has been cleaned. It is made by soaking and cooking the whole wheat kernel, drying it and then removing part of the bran and cracking the remaining kernels into small pieces. It then can be used in salads, soups, for breakfast and desserts. It is nutritional. It has a wide range of B vitamins. The grains provide iron, calcium, phosphorous, potassium, magnesium and zinc.
Coriander	Is parsley like in appearance. It is a spice made from the seeds of the cilantro plant. It is a light fresh flavor tinged with lemon. Its value is high in nutrition.
Jicama	Is a root crop that is grown from a vine. It is a sweet crispy edible root that resembles a turnip. Jicama has high fiber and is a delicious vegetable. It has the texture of water chestnuts. It is high in carbohydrates and it is in the form of dieting fiber.

Cardamon	Are aromatic seeds used as seasoning. It is within the ginger family. It has a spicy sweet pungent aroma. It is used in cakes, cookies, curries, fruit and Indian recipes.
Nutritional Yeast (Red Star®)	Is a terrific food, providing nutrition, enhancing flavor and adding taste to your favorite meals and drinks. It has an excellent source of protein, 52% containing essential amino acids. It is gluten free, rich in vitamins specially the B-complex vitamins. It is also an excellent source of folic acid, which is important for formation, growth and reproduction of red blood cells. It is commonly known as T6635T vegetarian support formula. The yeast is grown from pure strains of Saccharomyces Cerevisiae, grown on mixtures of cane and beets. Candida yeast infection (Candida Albicans), is a body yeast infection. Red Star® nutritional yeast (Saccharomyces Cerevisiae) is not found to be a cause of yeast or candida infection.
Sucanat	Is a contreaction of "sugare cane natural" or dark brown soft surgar. It is non-refined cane sugar, unlike refined and processed white sugar.

Resources

Reader's Digest Project Staff, Fight Back with Food, Pleasantville, NY 2002

George D. Pamplona-Roger, M. D., Education and Health Library, Foods and their Healing Power, (A Guide to Food Science and their Therapy). Review and Herald Publishing Association, USA and Canada Association 2004

E.G. White, Ministry of Healing, Health and Happiness, Better Living Publication, cooperation with Review and Herald and Pacific Press, USA 2002 Counsels on Health, Medical Missionary, Pacific Press, Publishing, Mountain View, CA. 1951

Dr. Antonia Demas, The Appleton School Project, Foods Grades & Behavior, Produced by Natural Ovens Bakery, Wisconsin, 1999

Hans A Diehl, Dr.HSe, MPH, Lifestyle Medicine, Lecture College of Medicine, Clinical Professor of Preventive Medicine Institute, Loma Linda, CA. 2004

Neal Bernard, MD., Food for Life, New York, New York Crown Publishers, 1995

Neil Nedley, MD Depression Recovery Program, Achieving peace of mind, restoring Energy to your Life, Nedley Publishing, Ardmore, Ok. 2005

Paul C. Bragg, N.D., PhD, Patricia Bragg, N.D., PhD, Healthful Eating without Confusion, Santa Barbara, California, 1999 - 2009

Dr. George Malkmus, Why Christians Get Sick, Shippensburg, Pennsylvania, Destiny Image, Inc., 1995

Agatha Thrash, M.D., Home Remedies, Yucchi Pines Institute, Seale, AL 1981

Dr. Ann Wigmore, Recipes for Longer Life, Wayne, New Jersey, Avery Publishing Group, Inc., 1978

Jean Carper, The Food Pharmacy, Dramatic New Evidence that Food is Your Best Medicine, (Featuring a pharmacopoeia of More than fifty foods.) Published by Bantam Books, New York, 1988

Dr. McDougall's Medicine, Diet VS Drugs, Director of the 10-day live-in McDougal Program in Santa Rosa Santa, California. 2007 DVD 14 Practical Cooking Demonstration Lessons from John and Mary McDougall.

European Commission's Joint Research Centre (JRC), preventing contamination of organic foods: http://online.sfsu.edu/-rone/GEessays/GMfree5.htm

Good Sprout News: http://www.isga-sprouts.org/history

Index

Breads and Crackers

- Amaranth Cereal 95
- Basic Whole Wheat Bread 95
- Fruity Nutty Granola 96
- Hardy Grain Cereal 97
- Oatmeal Apple Pancakes 97
- Pastry Wheat Raisin Nut Pancakes 98
- Sun Seed Crackers 98
- Wholesome Grain Crackers 99

Dairy Alternatives

- Cheesy Pimento Cashew Sauce 132
- Coconut Butter 131
- Dairy Free Butter 132
- Fruity Butter Spread 133
- Hummus Three in One 133
- Italian Tomato Sauce 134
- Jalapeno Tofu Cheese 134
- Non-Dairy Cottage Cheese 135
- Olive Butter 136
- Rice Cheese Spread 137
- Roasted Red Pepper Spread 137
- Spinach Dip Blend 138
- Thai Peanut Sauce 138
- The Best Mayonnaise 139

Delightful Pasta Dishes

- Artichoke Pesto Pasta 83
- Curried Penne 83
- Home Made Spaghetti with Sauce 84
- Meatless Lasagna 85
- Pasta and Chard 85
- Wheat Noodles with Walnuts 86

Eating more Raw for a Healthier Life

- Carrot Latte Soup 115
- Corn Chowder Soup 116
- Fennel Salad Combo 117
- Gazpacho Power Soup 117
- Green Life Soup 118
- Healthy Creamy Coleslaw 119
- Life Thriving Soup 120
- Mellon Soup 120
- Nutty Loaf 121
- Quinoa Veggie Mix 121

Guiltless Desserts

- Apple Cake 103
- Apricot Cake 103
- Banana Cream Pie 104
- Carrot Cake 105
- Frozen Fruit Dessert 107
- Fruit Squares 106
- Strawberry Biscuit Torte 108
- The Whole Apple Pie 109
- Tropical Fruitcake 110
- Yammy Pecan Mini Tarts 111

Herbal Seasonings

- Aromatic Veggie Seasoning 149
- Chili Powder 149
- Curry Powder 149
- Italian Seasoning 149
- Savory Vegetable Seasoning 150
- Veggie Chicken - Style Seasoning 150

Juicing For Life

- Brain Tonic Malt 125
- Cleansing Remedy 125
- Energy Boost Smoothie 125
- Green Smoothies 126
- Mid-Day Boost 126
- Nourishing Drink 127
- Peachy Cream 127
- Power House Fruit Smoothie 127
- Springaide 128
- Sprouting Life 128
- Yammy Veggie 128

Salad Dressings

- Creamy Garlic and Onion Salad Dressing 55
- Italian Dressing 55
- Pimento Relish Dressing 55
- Sesame Seed Dressing 56
- Sour Cream Dressing 56
- Thousand Island dressing 56
- Tomato Almond Dressing 57

Satisfying Rice Dishes

- Brown Rice with Cranberries 88
- Spanish Brown Rice 89
- Tofu Fry with Potatoes and Rice 89
- Vegetable Style Brown Rice 90
- Wild Rice Fiesta with Lentils and Tortilla Strips ... 91
- Wild Rice Pilaf with Vegetables 92
- Wild Rice with Butternut 92

Scrumptious Salads

- Black Bean Salad 45
- Cabbage Salad 45

Index (cont.)

Fruit Salad Mix 46
Garbanzo Bean Salad 47
Green Bean Salad 48
Green Vegetable Salad 49
Kidney Bean Avocado Salad 50
Potato Cucumber Salad 51
Tabbouleh 52

Tasty Soups And Stews

Black Bean Chili 61
Black French Lentil Soup 62
Cabbage Corn Chowder 62
Chili Pinto Beans 63
Cream of Asparagus Soup 64
Creamy Broccoli Chowder 65
Greek White Bean Soup 65
Lentil Combo 66
Northern Bean Soup 67
Potato Vegetable Soup 67
Savory Chickpea Stew 68
Tomato Tofu Soup 69

Vegetables And Entrée Dishes

Asparagus with Cream Sauce 73
Broccoli Tofu Scramble 74
Cheesy Broccoli 75
Creamy Spinach with Rice Cheese 76
Fancy Brussels Sprouts 75
Herb Roasted Vegetables 77
Honey Carrots 77
Mock Cottage Cheese Loaf 78
Pecan Loaf 78
Sugar Peas with Carrots 79
Tasty Greens 79

About the Author

Juanita Prince's motivation for an interest in healthy nutrition began when growing up as a child. Her mother was constantly seeking ways to educate and nourish her children well, so she sent them to private schools, which were Monterey Bay Academy and Pacific Union College. At that time she pursued an education in Nursing, Life Skills and nutrition.

After completing her education, she received a BA in Family Science with an emphasis in nutrition from Cal Poly in San Luis Obispo, California and a Master's in Education from Azusa Pacific University, California.

She was hired to teach Nutrition and other subjects at Fremont Junior High School in California for over twenty years. Her classroom was set up with six kitchens, where she taught young people the benefits of good health.

Juanita was not confined to her classroom; she shared and used her skills with others as well. She was interviewed on Jones Cable TV in Oxnard California. She was also placed in the Spokesman Review on front page of the of the food section twice in Spokane, Washington. Her other involvements included health fairs, healthy food demos in the community, the Farmer's Market and health food stores. She also prepares nutritious meals for churches and special events.

After leaving Southern California and moving to Washington State, she continued her work. She taught nutrition classes in both middle school and high school. She became actively involved in the community as a regional director for a large program called CHIP (Coronary Health Project), which was founded and directed by Han Diehl, Dr.H.Sc., at the Lifestyle Medicine Institute in Loma Linda, California. Juanita believes that a labor of love, is loving others, and teaching them good health principles, by preparing holistic nutritional meals to maintain a healthy body.

Her book offers the importance of taking care of one's own health, in the changing world that we live in. It offers insight why a plant diet is beneficial to a person and to the planet as well.

We invite you to view the complete
selection of titles we publish at:

www.LNFBooks.com

or write or email us your praises,
reactions, or thoughts about this
or any other book we publish at:

TEACH Services, Inc.
P.O. Box 954
Ringgold, GA 30736

info@TEACHServices.com

www.ingramcontent.com/pod-product-compliance
Lightning Source LLC
Chambersburg PA
CBHW070539170426
43200CB00011B/2473